KETOGENIC DIET FOR RAPID FAT LOSS AND WEIGHT LOSS

Everything You Need to Start a Ketogenic Diet Now, Including 50+ Fat Burning Recipes and an 8-Week Meal Plan

Janie Sanders

Digital Print House Inc

Table of Contents

Introduction

Most adults would like to lose some weight, but end up stuck in a cycle of crash dieting and regaining the weight. Does that sound familiar? No matter what diets you try, you always end up right back where you started a few months later. Maybe you are so overweight that no diet and exercise program seems to make a measurable difference. Even if you have managed to lose weight, do you still find yourself feeling sluggish in the afternoons? Are your cravings for sugary sweets keeping you from sticking to your diet? If any of these situations rings true, a ketogenic diet is for you. In this book, you will learn all about the revolutionary ketogenic diet and how to easily implement it in your life.

Of all the books and websites dedicated to ketogenic dieting, this one is unique; each of the 50+ recipes includes full nutritional information and suggestions on flavor variations so you will not feel stuck in a rut. This book includes an 8-week meal plan full of keto-friendly and delicious meals. The information in this book comes from countless hours of personal experience, including the experiences of hundreds of loyal ketogenic dieters.

Whether you have tried every diet under the sun or are just now starting your weight loss journey, this is the book for you. Once you start seeing results, you will not even miss the carbohydrates—especially because this book contains recipes for keto-friendly waffles, muffins, and milkshakes! Inside, you will find tips on how to navigate a ketogenic diet during social gatherings, what role snacks have in the diet, and how to shop for ketogenic-friendly foods on a budget. You will have more energy, fewer cravings, and more confidence as you commit to a ketogenic diet.

There is no better time to start than now.

The number of people who have discovered more energy and confidence through ketogenic dieting is growing. Are you finally ready to love your body and get out of the cycle of cravings and blood sugar crashes? Would you like to break your body's dependence on sugar and carbohydrates and start burning fat now? Keep reading to find everything you need to know about the ketogenic diet and how to start seeing benefits in your own life.

Chapter 1:
What Is a Ketogenic Diet?

"Ketogenic dieters report increased energy, focus, and remarkable weight loss results."

A ketogenic diet is a low-carb diet that pushes your body to derive energy from fat instead of from glucose. This metabolic process is called *ketosis*, and the goal of a ketogenic diet is to reach and maintain ketosis. A ketogenic diet can be beneficial for weight loss, building stamina, avoiding blood sugar crashes, and as part of treatment for diabetes or chronic fatigue. The ketogenic diet was first developed to treat epilepsy in children, although it became less popular as anticonvulsant drugs were developed. The name of the diet comes from the ketosis process.

Advantages of a Ketogenic Diet

One of the best things about a ketogenic diet is that there are no special foods needed to follow it. Many delicious foods restricted on other diets are fair game on a ketogenic diet. A few examples include bacon, butter, heavy cream, steak, and fried chicken. On the other hand, all grains and starchy vegetables are off limits, as are many fruits. A ketogenic diet is great for losing stubborn weight that has not come off with regular exercise. Ketogenic dieters often report increased energy and focus as well. When their bodies cease relying on glucose for energy, they avoid blood sugar spikes and drops that contribute to fatigue and sleepiness.

Warnings and Precautions

Like with any change in diet or lifestyle, transitioning to a ketogenic diet should be done carefully and under medical supervision. Some of the more common negative side effects include kidney stones, dehydration, and constipation.

Kidney Stones

Ketogenic dieters have a heightened risk of kidney stones if they eat too much protein relative to the rest of their diet. High levels of animal protein especially can contribute to kidney stones. Because many ketogenic diets are high in red meats and eggs, some people find themselves at risk of developing kidney stones. Calculating and sticking to the correct percentages of protein in your diet will reduce that risk. Another way to prevent kidney stones is to get more fat and protein from nuts to slightly reduce the amount of animal protein you consume. Proper hydration will also make it less likely that you develop a kidney stone.

Dehydration

Many ketogenic dieters, especially those new to the diet, report extreme thirst. Be sure to drink more water while on ketosis, especially if you feel thirsty. Any low-carb diet can lead to an electrolyte imbalance, so many ketogenic dieters treat both at the same time with sugar-free sports drinks or a good multivitamin. When looking for a vitamin or electrolyte replacement, be sure to account for sodium, chloride, potassium, calcium, and magnesium. Warm, homemade bone broth is a savory and nutritious meal replacement or supplement that also combats dehydration. When you begin a ketogenic diet, be sure to have plenty of water and bone broth available so you will not get dehydrated. This is especially important if you are spending time in hot weather or exercising.

Constipation

Because a ketogenic diet restricts grain and fruit consumption, many dieters find themselves with varying levels of constipation. Fortunately, the situation can be remedied by staying properly hydrated and eating more leafy, green vegetables. Other dieters keep laxatives handy just in case. Consuming extra magnesium can have a similar effect. If the constipation is not uncomfortable, it may not even be a problem; a ketogenic diet will inherently produce less waste. What some dieters assume is constipation is often just a less-regular bowel movement.

Chapter 1 Takeaways

1. Ketosis is a metabolic process that drives the body to burn fat for energy instead of burning glucose.

2. While on ketosis, you can experience rapid weight loss, improved stamina, and increased energy.

3. A ketogenic diet does not require any specialty foods; it can be followed with simple, nutritious staples from your neighborhood grocery store.

4. As always, consult a medical professional if you have any concerns.

Chapter 2:
Ketogenic Diet Myths

"As you become familiar with the main tenets of a ketogenic diet, you will be able to customize it to fit your lifestyle and needs."

A number of myths exist about the ketogenic diet. Many of these myths come from word-of-mouth or misunderstandings about various aspects of a ketogenic diet. Some of the most common myths are identified and explained below.

Myth #1: A Ketogenic Diet Is Only Safe Short-Term

Some critics of ketogenic diets claim that they are only safe short-term. In fact, a 2004 study by Dashti et al. studying the long-term effects of a ketogenic diet found no higher danger to the patients at 24 weeks than at the beginning of the diet.[1] As long as you are following basic safety precautions, a ketogenic diet can be a safe option long-term. If you are concerned about any general or specific health risks, consider having blood work done every 6-12 months. Your doctor can run a panel of tests on your blood and let you know if you need any additional vitamin supplements. Many ketogenic dieters find that their blood work results show them healthier than ever, often due to the fact that they are able to lose so much unhealthy weight.

---

[1] Dashti HM, Matthew TC, Hussein T, Asfar SK, Behbahani A, Khoursheed MA, Al-Sayer HM, Bo-Abbas YY & Al-Zaid NS (2004) Long-term effects of a ketogenic diet in obese patients. Exp Clin Cardiol 9:200-205.

Myth #2: A Ketogenic Diet Is the Same Thing as a Paleo Diet

There are many similarities between ketogenic and paleo diets. Both diets eliminate refined sugars, grains, and beans. There are many significant differences between the diets, however. A ketogenic diet is all about getting the body into ketosis. For this reason, most fruits are off limits. A paleo diet does not include dairy and can be high in carbohydrates from fruits and starchy vegetables. Some paleo diets are low-carb, but they are not always ketogenic. It is possible to follow both diets at once. Because of the similarities between some parts of the diet, many paleo recipes can also be easily modified for a ketogenic diet.

Myth #3: Athletes and Active Adults Cannot Follow a Ketogenic Diet

This myth stems from the idea that athletes cannot gain muscle mass on a low-carb diet. Even with the widespread nature of that assumption, athletes around the world are turning to ketogenic diets. There are many possible reasons for this. For starters, a ketogenic diet increases stamina and endurance. Another benefit that attracts professional and amateur athletes to a ketogenic diet is how it helps keep weight down. Slimming down helps many athletes perform better and feel stronger. In 2014, SI.com reported that LeBron James had been using a ketogenic diet during the off-season with the blessing of his doctor.[2]

---

[2] Lisanti, Jamie, "Inside LeBron James' Weight Loss and Low-Carb Diet," *Sports Illustrated,* August 11 2014, http://www.si.com/edge/2014/08/11/inside-lebron-james-weight-loss-and-low-carb-diet.

There are some basic modifications you can make to your ketogenic diet when you are attempting to gain muscle mass. First, you may need to reduce your workout schedule for the first two weeks on the diet. Some new ketogenic dieters experience a transition period of one to two weeks. During this period, you may have less energy and endurance than before. Once you make it past the transition (sometimes called "keto flu"), you will be able to increase the intensity of your workouts back to normal. When working out on a ketogenic diet during and after the transition, be sure to drink plenty of water. You may also find it helpful to occasionally increase your calorie and/or carbohydrate intake very slightly immediately before a workout if you are attempting to bulk up.

Myth #4: Ketogenic Diets Are One-Size-Fits-All

The basics of ketogenic diets are simple, but the implementation varies from person to person. Some dieters choose to eat only unprocessed, natural foods. Others embrace the many low-carb supplements and ingredients on the market. Some dieters embrace intermittent fasting days, starting the day with Bulletproof Coffee (pg. 56) or Bone Broth (pg. 116) and not eating again until a small meal in the evening. The general recommendation for ketogenic diets is to keep carbohydrate consumption under 50g daily. Other keto dieters find better results closer to 20-30g carbohydrates each day. As you become familiar with the main tenets of a ketogenic diet, you will be able to customize it to fit your lifestyle and needs.

Chapter 2 Takeaways

1. Studies show that a ketogenic diet can be safe long-term.

2. While a paleo diet and a ketogenic diet have many things in common, they are not the same. It is possible (but not necessary) to follow a diet that is both paleo- and keto-friendly.

3. A ketogenic diet can be successful for athletes. Some professional sports teams are even using the diet as a team.

4. A ketogenic diet is flexible enough to be adapted to fit your preferences and needs.

Chapter 3:
Why It Works

"A ketogenic diet works because it trains your body to burn fat instead of glucose."

Ketogenic dieting can seem complicated at first, primarily because it relies so much on accurately keeping track of what you eat. The main component of any ketogenic diet, however, is ketosis. Once you understand ketosis, the rest will be easier to remember.

Understanding Ketosis

Your body gets energy from breaking down bonds in the foods you eat. Because glucose is the easiest type of food for the body to convert to energy, it will naturally break down glucose before fats or proteins. On a traditional diet, glucose is the main source of energy. When the body cannot get all of its energy from glucose, it will next turn to breaking down fat. Ketosis is the name of the metabolic process when the body gets energy from fat instead of glucose. The name comes from chemicals called ketones, which are released from the liver during ketosis.

It is important to know that ketosis is not the same thing as *diabetic ketoacidosis* (DKA). The former simply refers to the body deriving energy from fat (both consumed and stored in the body). DKA is a dangerous condition that sometimes affects Type 1 diabetics due to insulin deficiency. The ketosis activated by a ketogenic diet is not the same thing and does not carry the same fatal risks because ketone levels are much higher in DKA than in nutritional ketosis.

How a Ketogenic Diet Affects the Body

Some people find the transition to a ketogenic diet takes a full two weeks. Those who have a difficult transition describe it as "keto flu": exhaustion, body aches, and extreme thirst. Many new dieters do not experience any negative symptoms at all. Consuming enough electrolytes, increasing sodium intake temporarily, and staying hydrated are suggested methods for avoiding a difficult transition.

Once your body has adjusted to ketosis, you will experience any number of beneficial effects. A ketogenic diet is more satiating than a traditional diet; you will feel full longer and experience fewer cravings throughout the day. Most ketogenic dieters report higher energy, clearer skin, and more mental clarity on ketosis. As mentioned in the beginning of this book, the ketogenic diet has been used for decades to treat certain types of epilepsy. Chronic fatigue symptoms and causes vary by patient, but many find that reducing carbohydrate intake produces positive results. Other medical conditions that can be treated (in part) with a ketogenic diet include PCOS and type 2 diabetes.[3]

Losing Weight on a Ketogenic Diet

One of the main reasons people love the ketogenic diet is because it leads to incredibly effective weight loss. It is important to avoid overconsumption of carbohydrates when trying to shed extra pounds. Dietary glucose comes from carbohydrates. When the body is relying on glucose for energy, it will store any extra glucose as fat. By extension, overconsumption of carbohydrates results in the body stockpiling more and more fat for later use.

---

[3] Yancy WS, Jr, Foy M, Chalecki AM, Vernon MC & Westman EC (2005) A low-carbohydrate, ketogenic diet to treat type 2 diabetes. Nutr Metab (Lond) 2:34.

A daily ketogenic menu should contain fewer than 50 grams carbohydrates. Dramatically reducing the number of carbohydrates you consume will force your body into ketosis. Once in ketosis, your body will derive energy from fat—including any extra fat stores you already have! This is the main reason for weight loss on a ketogenic diet. You are training your body to burn fat instead of saving it for later.

Some dieters may find that they need to reduce their carbohydrate intake even further to enter ketosis, but <50g is a common daily goal. Especially when starting out, the carbohydrate count is the number that matters most. If you are not losing weight as fast as you would like on a ketogenic diet, it may be necessary to also track your calories. The most important thing is transitioning your body to ketosis so that it will begin to rely on dietary and stored fat for energy.

Many ketogenic dieters count net carbohydrates instead of total carbohydrates. Net carbohydrates are calculated by calculating total carbohydrates minus dietary fiber. The recipes in this book give total carbohydrates for simplicity's sake, except when there is a significant difference between the two (as with any recipe containing flax seed meal or chia seeds).

Chapter 3 Takeaways

1. When your body enters ketosis, it will use up fat stores for energy.

2. Ketosis is not the same thing as diabetic ketoacidosis.

3. You can avoid or reduce the effects of "keto flu" by staying hydrated and increasing your sodium intake the first week on a ketogenic diet.

4. After a transition period, a ketogenic diet can lead to better-looking skin, weight loss, and more energy.

5. A ketogenic diet should contain no more than 50g of carbohydrates per day. Some dieters reduce this number to 30g, while others calculate net carbohydrates (carbohydrates minus dietary fiber).

6. You should consume as much fat as necessary to feel full and satisfied.

Chapter 4:
Is a Ketogenic Diet Right for You?

"A ketogenic diet is more satisfying and can cost less than what you are eating now."

After reading all about the benefits of a ketogenic diet, you are probably ready to begin the process yourself. It is not a diet that can be done half-heartedly. To be most successful, a ketogenic diet must be a complete commitment. The benefits are numerous, however, and well worth the effort. Making the transition to a ketogenic diet is often the hardest part. Once you are accustomed to a ketogenic diet and have started to see results, it will be easier to stick with it. In this chapter, you will learn how to implement a ketogenic diet in your life easily and effectively.

How to Easily Make the Transition to a Ketogenic Diet

One easy way to transition to a ketogenic diet is to start by making your regular meals keto-friendly. Instead of spaghetti and marinara sauce, eat meat sauce with cheese. Instead of eggs and toast, opt for a larger plate of eggs with bacon or ham. If your family is eating pot roast, simply leave out the traditional potatoes. Enjoy roast with pan drippings and a green salad instead.

Another important part of transitioning to a ketogenic diet is keeping track of what you consume. Invest in a kitchen scale and track your intake. After a few weeks, it will become second nature to calculate the nutritional information of your meals. If you end up needing to make any adjustments to your diet, you can turn to your records and easily see trends that may need changing. When you plan, aim for 50g carbohydrates or fewer each day. At least 60% of your daily calories should come from fat. Many ketogenic dieters find a high-quality multivitamin vital in reaching nutritional goals without going over the daily carbohydrate limit.

When you shop, be sure to carefully read the label of any prepared foods or condiments. There is great variation from brand to brand, especially in sugar and carbohydrates. Some products are marketed specifically as no-sugar or low-carb, but even the meaning of these labels can vary from brand to brand.

Helpful Resources

When you are transitioning to a ketogenic diet, you may find it difficult to keep track of your carbohydrate and fat consumption. You may wonder if you are actually entering and maintaining ketosis. You may want to adapt treasured family recipes to be keto-friendly. Fortunately, there are all kinds of resources available for each of these goals.

Ketone test strips can be purchased online or at a local pharmacy near the diabetes supplies. These test strips change color when exposed to ketones in urine. Following the directions on the package, you will be able to test your ketones and figure out if you are currently in ketosis. In time, you will recognize the characteristics of ketosis and be able to identify it without ketone strips.

Two websites regularly used by ketogenic dieters to figure out calorie distribution and dietary goals are My Fitness Pal (myfitnesspal.com) and Keto Calculator (keto-calculator.ankerl.com), although many other websites and forums are also dedicated to aiding ketogenic diets. Calculating nutritional information of recipes is relatively simple, with a number of websites and apps dedicated to that purpose, allowing you to simply input ingredients and quantities to calculate the calories, fat, protein, vitamins, and carbohydrates of your favorite recipes. You can even adjust the number of servings to see how the values change based on how many meals you make out of any specific recipe. For the purposes of this book, nutritional information was calculated with Spark Recipes (recipes.sparkpeople.com). Other popular resources include Fit Day (fitday.com) and SELF Nutrition Data (nutritiondata.self.com).

Ketogenic Diet on a Budget

At first glance, a ketogenic diet may appear to be an expensive endeavor. Meat and seafood, especially the grass-fed and wild-caught varieties, can be much more expensive than packaged foods high in carbohydrates and fillers. A shopper accustomed to purchasing regular milk may balk at the price tag on heavy cream or full-fat yogurt. In reality, a ketogenic diet often costs *less* than a more mainstream one. You will eat less food when you are eating nutrient- and fat-dense foods. The elimination of mindless grazing and snacking will actually lower your grocery bill over time. That being said, there are still times you may need to watch your food budget closely. Whether you are just starting out or find yourself in a tight month financially, here are some tested methods for keeping food costs down on a ketogenic diet:

Shop the Sales

The 8-week meal plan included at the end of this book is a great resource for planning a diverse rotation of meals. There may be a week when you plan to eat Slow Cooker Pot Roast (pg. 90) and find another cut of meat on sale instead. For example, pork shoulder makes a delicious slow cooker roast as well. Trout en Papillote (pg. 75) is equally tasty made from any flaky, white fish; other acceptable varieties include catfish, cod, tilapia, and snapper. Other easy substitutions include types of cheese, chicken thighs for chicken breasts, and ground turkey or pork for ground beef.

As you become more familiar with the recipes you like, it will be easier to spot a great deal. Swapping out one meat for another is one of the easiest ways to take advantage of sales, because meat is likely to make up a large portion of your grocery bill each week. If you do find a favorite cut of meat on sale, stock up! Most meat freezes beautifully for at least six months.

Plan Simple Meals

The beauty of a ketogenic diet is that both a T-bone steak with eggs and a cup of Bulletproof Coffee (pg. 56) are keto-friendly meals. There is a wide range of complexities when it comes to meal options. Planning simpler meals occasionally can keep food costs down.

Eggs are a relatively inexpensive source of protein and fat. Hard-boiled eggs make a great snack or addition to a meal. In addition to breakfast, consider having scrambled or fried eggs for dinner. With shredded cheese and a half an avocado, a plate of scrambled eggs can be a satisfying and inexpensive meal. Most stores sell eggs in bulk (up to six dozen at a time), making it even easier to stock up on this incredible protein.

Bone broth is a nutrient-dense staple in any ketogenic pantry. In addition to use in soups and sauces, bone broth is a delicious meal by itself. As your body detoxes off of extra sugars and carbohydrates, you will find yourself satisfied by smaller meals. A warm cup of bone broth is a perfect (and delicious) meal on days when other meals will be heavier or take more preparation.

Buy in Bulk

Once you know what meals fit your time and tastes, you can begin to buy common ingredients in bulk. Freezing individual servings of meat from a larger purchase will save money and allow you to control portion size. Freezing is also a good option for berries, grapes, and other fruit. Because fruit should be consumed sparingly on a ketogenic diet, you may find you cannot eat an entire container before it spoils. Frozen berries, grapes, and cherries make delicious snacks. Just a few bites will cool you down and satisfy any cravings for something juicy and sweet.

Buy Specialty Ingredients over Time

There are many specialty low-carb products on the market, especially for baking. Low- or no-carb protein powders and shakes, nut flours, no-sugar sweeteners, and baking aids like xantham gum can make it easier to recreate favorite foods in a keto-friendly way. However, it can be expensive to fill a pantry with supplements and specialty baking ingredients. Start with simple ingredients and purchase just one specialty item each week. It will take longer to stock your pantry that way, but it will be easier on your pocketbook. It will also give you a chance to become familiar with each new ingredient one at a time. With so many specialty items you may not have ever used before, you will get the most value out of your money spent if you are comfortable using them.

Chapter 4 Takeaways

1. A successful ketogenic diet requires a total commitment.

2. You can begin keto-friendly eating now by eliminating carbohydrates from the foods you already eat.

3. Having a plan and accurately tracking your daily meals are incredibly important.

4. A digital kitchen scale is an invaluable tool for measuring portions.

5. The internet is full of forums, websites, and apps dedicated to supporting your ketogenic diet.

6. By shopping sales and planning simple meals, a ketogenic diet can actually cost less than your current grocery budget.

7. Be sure to check the labels of prepared foods and condiments; not all low-carb products are created equal.

Chapter 5:
Common Ketogenic Diet Mistakes and How to Avoid Them

"The very best thing you can do to achieve success on a ketogenic diet is to make a plan."

While the tenets of a ketogenic diet are relatively simple, those new to the diet often make the same mistakes. The following four mistakes are common among new ketogenic dieters but can be easily avoided with a few simple steps.

Avoiding Fat

Your body will get energy from fat while on ketosis. It is very important that you eat enough healthy fats to maintain maximum energy and stamina. As an added bonus, a diet full of healthy fats will keep you full and satisfied longer after each meal. Many ketogenic dieters discover that they naturally eat less because they are not as hungry or subject to as many cravings, both of which are byproducts of eating enough fat. At least 60% of your daily calories should come from fat.

Once you've committed yourself to a ketogenic diet, you will have to train yourself not to avoid fat. Buy full-fat dairy products and condiments. Leave the skin on when you cook chicken (it will be tastier that way anyway), and use plenty of fat when you sauté or pan-fry vegetables or meats. If you are still struggling to get enough fat, start the day with a cup of Bulletproof Coffee (pg. 56). The early boost of fat will keep you full through the morning, and because Bulletproof Coffee has 0.0g carbohydrates per serving, it will not derail your nutritional goals for the day.

Forgetting About Drinks

Soft drinks, juice, and milk are extremely high in carbohydrates. The easiest way to avoid accidentally going over your carbohydrate limit is to simply stop drinking anything but water. There are many ketosis-friendly drinks, some of which are included in Chapter 8, but they should be carefully accounted for in your daily plan.

While some alcohols are acceptable from a ketosis standpoint, most beer, wine coolers, and mixed drinks are loaded with sugar and carbohydrates. Ketosis will also lower your tolerance to alcohol, so drink carefully and sparingly until you become accustomed to the change. You are likely to find that it takes many fewer drinks than usual to leave you feeling woozy. Hangovers can also be much worse during ketosis because it is easier to become dehydrated. You should always be drinking plenty of water on a ketogenic diet, but that is especially true during and after any alcohol consumption. Alternate drinks of water with sips of alcohol. Intentionally keeping hydrated will minimize the pain the next morning.

Even when you are not drinking alcohol, it is important to stay hydrated. A ketogenic diet can be dehydrating; your body will need much more water than usual. Make a habit of drinking water throughout the day: first thing in the morning, right after a shower, mid-afternoon, or when you get home from work. Soon you will be drinking extra water without much effort.

Not Making a Plan

The very best thing you can do to achieve success on a ketogenic diet is to make a plan and stick with it. Plan your meals, especially if you will be eating out or in a group. Once you get accustomed to packing your lunch, planning for social situations, and making decisions about snacks ahead of time, your ketogenic diet will be more successful. Don't forget the kitchen scale, which simplifies the process of measuring portions when calculating your daily totals. Small changes to your percentages and caloric intake can make a huge difference in your results, whether your goal is weight loss, muscle gain, or overall health. You will be better able to adjust your personal diet if you have a plan and the ability to measure it.

Chapter 5 Takeaways

1. The most common mistakes made by new ketogenic dieters are avoiding fat, forgetting about drinks, and not making a plan.

2. At least 60% of your daily caloric intake should come from fat.

3. It takes less alcohol on a ketogenic diet to feel the effects. It is also easier to get dehydrated. You can avoid painful hangovers by consuming water while you drink.

4. Sticking to your plan will guarantee your success!

Chapter 6:

What to Eat and What to Avoid

"A ketogenic diet is rich in meat, dairy, eggs, and vegetables."

The first goal on a ketogenic diet is to avoid unnecessary carbohydrates. To do this, remove added sugar from your diet, both from granulated sugar as well as honey, syrups or fruit juices. Even some fresh fruits are too high in natural sugars to be compatible with a ketogenic diet. The fruits that are highest in natural sugars (and carbohydrates) are pineapple, mango, cantaloupe, grapes, bananas, and kiwi. All dried fruits are extremely high in sugar and should be avoided. Wheat, oats, rice, and corn are almost completely off limits. Starchy potatoes (both white, yellow, and sweet) should also be avoided.

It may seem like many foods are off limits, but most unprocessed meats, eggs, dairy, and vegetables are all welcome components of a ketogenic diet. Even fresh berries have a place, as long as they serve as an occasional treat and not a major source of calories or carbohydrates. The best thing you can do for your ketogenic diet is stock up on high-quality meats and leafy greens. Grass-fed or pastured meats will taste better and be more nutritious. The same is true for wild-caught seafood. Butter and cream from grass-fed cows and eggs from free-range chickens have so much more flavor than their factory counterparts. Milk is much higher in carbohydrates per serving than heavy cream, so opt for cream instead. Small servings of fresh raspberries, blackberries, and strawberries can be a part of a ketogenic diet in moderation.

Fresh herbs and high-quality spices can really shine on a ketogenic diet. As you detox from the excessive sugar in your previous diet, you will find the natural sweetness in many foods is enough. Other spices will begin to taste better and you may find yourself experimenting with new combinations and flavors. A little goes a long way with dried herbs, and spending a little extra for better quality is worth the cost.

Best Foods to Keep On Hand

In addition to high-quality meats and seafood, there are a number of foods you should try to always have at home. These ingredients are common components in many ketogenic recipes. Making sure to keep them on hand will simplify meal preparation and keep you from grabbing something easy but loaded with carbohydrates. Add the following items to your grocery list to keep the pantry stocked with important staples:

Proteins
- Bacon
- Eggs
- Grass-fed beef
- Wild-caught fish
- Canned tuna and salmon
- Pastured pork and chicken
- Raw or low-salt roasted nuts

Dairy/Non-Dairy Milk Products
- Cream cheese
- Full-fat cheeses
- 4% milk fat cottage cheese
- Heavy cream
- Full-fat plain yogurt
- Unsweetened vanilla almond milk

- Coconut milk (both the canned milk in the Asian foods aisle and the refrigerated milk substitute)

Produce
- Leafy green vegetables (Swiss chard, kale, etc.)
- Celery
- Carrots
- Avocado
- Fresh garlic
- Cauliflower
- Fresh berries
- Cucumber
- Onions
- Spaghetti squash
- Fresh parsley
- Button mushrooms

Baking Supplies
- Almond flour and/or coconut flour
- Flax seed meal
- Chia seeds
- Xantham gum
- MCT oil
- Organic coconut oil
- Stevia powder or another low-carbohydrate sweetener

Condiments/Miscellaneous
- Homemade bone broth (pg. 116)
- Low-sugar ketchup*
- Natural peanut butter*
- Sugar-free flavoring syrups*
- Vanilla protein powder*
- Pork rinds/chicharrones

- Low-carb protein or snack bars*
- Black olives
- Xantham gum

*These products can vary quite a bit by brand. Be sure to check the labels for ingredients and values. Some brands are very ketosis-friendly, while others are loaded with added sugars.

Do You Need a Calorie Count?

At its most basic, a ketogenic diet is about restricting carbohydrates in order to encourage your body to enter ketosis. For this reason, most ketogenic diet plans do not focus on calories other than in tracking macros. It is far more important to eat when you are hungry and learn to listen to what your body needs. If you are following a true ketogenic diet full of unprocessed fats and proteins, you should not need to count calories.

To be the most successful on a ketogenic diet, however, you will need to keep careful track of what you consume. The longer you follow a ketogenic diet, the more intuitive your daily macros will become. When you are starting out, however, it is important to make sure you are getting enough of what you need (and not too much of anything else). Counting calories is a small part of this tracking process. Some new dieters find that they are eating diets high in fat *and* high in calories because they allow themselves cheat days. If you find yourself stalling in your weight loss or struggling to maintain ketosis, it may be worth the time and effort to count calories. Caloric intake should not be your primary concern on a ketogenic diet, but tracking your intake can help you get a better idea of what you are actually eating. It may be necessary to make a slight adjustment to daily caloric intake if needed.

Chapter 6 Takeaways

1. Eliminate all bread, grains, pastas, rice, and starchy vegetables from your diet.

2. Eat all you want of meats, eggs, green vegetables, and seafood.

3. Eat full-fat dairy products and cheese as long as you do not exceed your daily carbohydrate totals.

4. Buy high-quality fresh and dried herbs and use them liberally.

5. Protein powder or pork rinds can substitute for breadcrumbs or flour in some recipes.

6. When using xantham gum to thicken a recipe, remember that a little goes a long way!

7. You only need to count calories to get a feel for your daily totals. As long as you are remaining in ketosis and seeing the results you want, calories do not matter.

Chapter 7:

8-Week Meal Plan

"Our easy-to-follow meal plan will simplify the first two months of your ketogenic diet."

For the purposes of this meal plan, each day's target is 50g carbohydrates or less. Some days are even lower in carbohydrates, but all are under 50g total. Two snacks of no more than 5g net carbohydrates each are factored into the daily total. This can be two small snacks throughout the day, one larger snack in the afternoon, or 10g carbohydrates added to any single meal.

Feel free to enjoy any of the following snacks, all of which are under 5g net carbohydrates:

- 1/2 c. cottage cheese
- 4 medium radishes
- 1 celery stalk + 2 T. natural peanut butter
- 1/2 avocado
- 1/4 c. almonds
- 1/2 c. sliced cucumber
- 5-6 cherry tomatoes
- 1 stick string cheese + 5 black olives
- 2 boiled eggs
- 1/3 c. seedless grapes
- 1/2 c. fresh strawberries
- 1/4 c. pitted cherries
- 3 Ham and Cheese Pinwheel Roll Ups (pg. 111)
- 1/2 c. Kale Chips (pg. 107)
- 2 oz. summer sausage + 1/4 c. Chipotle Cheese Crackers (pg. 105)

- 2 Bacon-Wrapped Jalapeño Bites (pg. 110)
- 4 Deviled Eggs (pg. 108)

	Day 1	B: Baked Eggs and Corned Beef Hash + Bulletproof Coffee
		L: Curried Shrimp Soup
		D: Bacon-Wrapped Meatloaf + Creamed Spinach
	Day 2	B: Perfect 2-Egg Omelet + Strawberries and Cream Smoothie
		L: Chipotle Cheese Crackers + Caprese Salad
		D: Chicken Liver & Onions + Oven-Roasted Brussels Sprouts
	Day 3	B: Scrambled Eggs with Ham + Iced Green Tea
		L: Chicken Salad with Avocado
Week 1		D: Pork and Green Bean Stir Fry + Cauliflower "Rice"
	Day 4	B: Coconut Zucchini Muffin + Pumpkin Spice Smoothie
		L: Trout en Papillote + Grilled Mushroom Skewers
		D: Steak with Chimichurri Sauce + Bacon-Wrapped Asparagus
	Day 5	B: Vanilla Almond Waffle + Bulletproof Coffee
		L: Curried Egg Salad
		D: Spaghetti Squash with Meaty Marinara
	Day 6	B: Chocolate Peanut Butter Smoothie
		L: Chicken Sausage and Kale Soup
		D: Slow Cooker Pot Roast + Mashed

Cauliflower Puree

B: Overnight Chia Pudding

Day 7   L: Crunchy Chicken Strips + Kale Chips

D: White Chicken Chili

B: Nut and Seed Biscuits + Cinnamon Almond Milk

Day 1   L: Warm Bone Broth

D: Garlic and Lemon Roast Chicken + Oven-Roasted Broccoli

B: Fiesta Sausage and Egg Sandwich + Bulletproof Coffee

Day 2   L: Caprese Salad + Bacon-Wrapped Asparagus

D: Curried Shrimp Soup

B: Spinach and Bacon Frittata

Day 3   L: Chicken Salad with Avocado

D: Bacon-Wrapped Meatloaf + Mashed Cauliflower Puree

B: 2 Chocolate Chip Protein Bites + Bulletproof Coffee

Week 2

Day 4   L: Bacon and Cheese Broccoli Soup

D: Chicken Piccata + Lemon-Garlic Swiss Chard

B: Baked Vanilla Custard

Day 5   L: Coconut Zucchini Muffin + Curried Egg Salad

D: Lemon Rosemary Chicken Soup

B: Warm Flax Cereal + Bulletproof Coffee

Day 6   L: Lox and Cream Cheese Boats

D: Tandoori-Style Grilled Chicken + Oven-Roasted Broccoli

Day 7   B: Scrambled Eggs and Ham + Iced Green Tea

Day 1	L: White Chicken Chili
	D: Pork and Green Bean Stir Fry + Cauliflower "Rice"
	B: Baked Eggs and Corned Beef Hash
	L: Crunchy Chicken Strips + Thick and Creamy Vanilla Shake
	D: Spaghetti Squash with Meaty Marinara + Green Salad
Day 2	B: Nut and Seed Biscuits +Pumpkin Spice Smoothie
	L: Warm Bone Broth
	D: Pork and Green Bean Stir Fry + Cauliflower "Rice"
Day 3	B: Perfect 2-Egg Omelet + Chocolate Peanut Butter Smoothie
	L: Chipotle Cheese Crackers + Bacon and Cheese Broccoli Soup
	D: Slow Cooker Pot Roast + Oven Roasted Asparagus
Day 4	B: Vanilla Almond Waffle + Bulletproof Coffee
	L: Chicken Salad with Avocado
	D: Steak with Chimichurri Sauce + Creamed Spinach
Day 5	B: Coconut Zucchini Muffin + Cinnamon Almond Milk
	L: Curried Shrimp Soup
	D: Spinach and Bacon Frittata + Green Salad
Day 6	B: Scrambled Eggs and Ham + Strawberries and Cream Smoothie
	L: Lemon Rosemary Chicken Soup
	D: Garlic and Lemon Roast Chicken + Oven-Roasted Broccoli

Week 3

	Day 7	B: Warm Flax Cereal + Bulletproof Coffee L: Lox and Cream Cheese Boats D: Chicken Liver & Onions + Grilled Mushroom Skewers
Week 4	Day 1	B: Overnight Chia Pudding + Bulletproof Coffee L: Chicken Sausage and Kale Soup D: Salmon Cakes + Oven-Roasted Broccoli
	Day 2	B: Fiesta Sausage and Egg Sandwich + Bulletproof Coffee L: Trout en Papillote + Green Salad D: Chicken Piccata + Lemon-Garlic Swiss Chard
	Day 3	B: Baked Vanilla Custard L: Crunchy Chicken Strips + Kale Chips D: Chicken Piccata + Caprese Salad
	Day 4	B: Scrambled Eggs with Ham + Iced Green Tea L: Chicken Salad with Avocado D: Pork and Green Bean Stir Fry + Cauliflower "Rice"
	Day 5	B: Warm Flax Cereal + Bulletproof Coffee L: Lox and Cream Cheese Boats D: Tandoori-Style Grilled Chicken + Oven-Roasted Broccoli
	Day 6	B: Coconut Zucchini Muffin + Cinnamon Almond Milk L: Curried Shrimp Soup D: Steak with Chimichurri Sauce + Creamed Spinach
	Day 7	B: Baked Eggs and Corned Beef Hash + Bulletproof Coffee L: Crunchy Chicken Strips + Thick and

		Creamy Vanilla Shake
		D: Spaghetti Squash with Meaty Marinara
	Day 1	B: Baked Vanilla Custard
		L: Coconut Zucchini Muffin + Warm Bone Broth
		D: Lemon Rosemary Chicken Soup
	Day 2	B: Fiesta Sausage and Egg Sandwich + Bulletproof Coffee
		L: Trout en Papillote + Oven-Roasted Brussels Sprouts
		D: Chicken Piccata + Lemon-Garlic Swiss Chard
	Day 3	B: Perfect 2-Egg Omelet + Chocolate Peanut Butter Smoothie
Week 5		L: Chipotle Cheese Crackers + Bacon and Cheese Broccoli Soup
		D: Slow Cooker Pot Roast
	Day 4	B: Warm Flax Cereal + Bulletproof Coffee
		L: Lox and Cream Cheese Boats
		D: Tandoori-Style Grilled Chicken + Oven-Roasted Broccoli
	Day 5	B: 2 Chocolate Chip Protein Bites + Bulletproof Coffee
		L: Bacon and Cheese Broccoli Soup
		D: Bacon-Wrapped Meatloaf + Mashed Cauliflower Puree
	Day 6	B: Scrambled Eggs with Ham + Strawberries and Cream Smoothie
		L: Chipotle Cheese Crackers + Caprese Salad
		D: Chicken Liver & Onions + Oven-Roasted Asparagus
	Day 7	B: Coconut Zucchini Muffin + Cinnamon Almond Milk

Week 6	Day 1	L: Curried Shrimp Soup D: Spinach and Bacon Frittata + Green Salad B: Vanilla Almond Waffle + Bulletproof Coffee L: Curried Egg Salad D: Spaghetti Squash with Meaty Marinara
	Day 2	B: Nut and Seed Biscuits + Cinnamon Almond Milk L: Salmon Cakes + Caprese Salad D: Garlic and Lemon Roast Chicken + Oven-Roasted Broccoli
	Day 3	B: Scrambled Eggs and Ham + Iced Green Tea L: White Chicken Chili D: Pork and Green Bean Stir Fry + Cauliflower "Rice"
	Day 4	B: Coconut Zucchini Muffin + Pumpkin Spice Smoothie L: Warm Bone Broth D: Steak with Chimichurri Sauce + Creamed Spinach
	Day 5	B: Warm Flax Cereal + Bulletproof Coffee L: Lox and Cream Cheese Boats D: Chicken Liver & Onions + Mashed Cauliflower Puree
	Day 6	B: Spinach and Bacon Frittata L: Chicken Salad with Avocado + Celery Spears D: Bacon-Wrapped Meatloaf + Thick and Creamy Vanilla Shake
	Day 7	B: Baked Eggs and Corned Beef Hash + Bulletproof Coffee L: Curried Shrimp Soup

		D: Bacon-Wrapped Meatloaf + Bacon-Wrapped Asparagus
	Day 1	B: Perfect 2-Egg Omelet + Chocolate Peanut Butter Smoothie
		L: Chipotle Cheese Crackers + Bacon and Cheese Broccoli Soup
		D: Slow Cooker Pot Roast
	Day 2	B: Fiesta Sausage and Egg Sandwich
		L: Trout en Papillote + Warm Bone Broth
		D: Chicken Piccata + Lemon-Garlic Swiss Chard
	Day 3	B: Perfect 2-Egg Omelet + Strawberries and Cream Smoothie
		L: Deviled Eggs + Green Salad
		D: Chicken Liver & Onions + Oven-Roasted Brussels Sprouts
Week 7	Day 4	B: Vanilla Almond Waffle + Bulletproof Coffee
		L: Curried Egg Salad
		D: Spaghetti Squash with Meaty Marinara
	Day 5	B: Spinach and Bacon Frittata
		L: Chicken Salad with Avocado + Celery Spears
		D: Bacon-Wrapped Meatloaf + Green Salad
	Day 6	B: Chocolate Peanut Butter Smoothie
		L: Chicken Sausage and Kale Soup
		D: Slow Cooker Pot Roast + Mashed Cauliflower Puree
	Day 7	B: Baked Vanilla Custard
		L: Coconut Zucchini Muffin + Curried Egg Salad
		D: Lemon Rosemary Chicken Soup

Week 8	Day 1	B: Warm Flax Cereal + Bulletproof Coffee L: Lox and Cream Cheese Boats D: Tandoori-Style Grilled Chicken + Oven-Roasted Broccoli
	Day 2	B: Nut and Seed Biscuits + Cinnamon Almond Milk L: Salmon Cakes D: Garlic and Lemon Roast Chicken + Bacon-Wrapped Asparagus
	Day 3	B: Scrambled Eggs with Ham + Iced Green Tea L: Chicken Salad with Avocado D: Pork and Green Bean Stir Fry + Cauliflower "Rice"
	Day 4	B: 2 Chocolate Chip Protein Bites + Bulletproof Coffee L: Bacon and Cheese Broccoli Soup D: Bacon-Wrapped Meatloaf + Mashed Cauliflower Puree
	Day 5	B: Coconut Zucchini Muffin + Pumpkin Spice Smoothie L: Warm Bone Broth D: Steak with Chimichurri Sauce + Creamed Spinach
	Day 6	B: Baked Eggs and Corned Beef Hash L: Crunchy Chicken Strips + Thick and Creamy Vanilla Shake D: Spaghetti Squash with Meaty Marinara
	Day 7	B: Vanilla Almond Waffle + Bulletproof Coffee L: Salmon Cakes + Kale Chips D: Spaghetti Squash with Meaty Marinara

Chapter 7 Takeaways

1. There are so many delicious ways to eat on a ketogenic diet. Use this diet plan to discover your favorite meal combinations.

2. If there is a meal that does not sound good to you, make substitutions as desired. The total nutritional information for each meal on the meal plan can be found in Chapter 8.

3. Make a list of snacks you enjoy that contain 5g carbohydrates or fewer. Keeping these snacks on hand will help curb any cravings you have for starchy or sweet snacks.

Chapter 8:

Top Ketogenic Recipes

"56 delicious and diverse recipes for your ketosis journey."

Breakfast

Baked Eggs and Corned Beef Hash

Prep Time: 5 minutes

Cook Time: 15 minutes

Yield: 6 servings

Ingredients:

1 T. extra virgin olive oil

1/2 c. chopped onion

1 green bell pepper, minced

2 cloves garlic, minced

1 lb. corned beef brisket, cubed

6 eggs

Directions:

Preheat oven to 375°F. Heat olive oil in a cast-iron skillet over medium-high heat. When the oil is shimmering, add the onion and pepper. Sauté until the onions are translucent. Stir in garlic and cook for 30 seconds, being careful not to let the garlic burn. Add corned beef and heat through.

Once the corned beef is hot, turn off the heat. Make 6 small depressions in the corned beef hash and crack 1 egg into each well. Bake for 8-10 minutes or until the eggs are cooked to the desired doneness.

Nutritional Information (per serving):
Calories: 293.2
Fat: 21.5 g
Cholesterol: 260.0 mg
Sodium: 928.4 mg
Potassium: 203.5 mg
Carbohydrate: 3.6 g
Protein: 20.4 g

Perfect 2-Egg Omelet

Prep Time: 5 minutes
Cook Time: 2 minutes
Yield: 1 omelet

Ingredients:
2 large eggs (fresh eggs are best)
2 tsp. unsalted butter, divided
1/4 tsp. kosher salt
1/2 T. chopped chives
2 T. shredded white cheddar cheese

Directions:
Whisk eggs together until smooth. There should be no discernable difference between egg yolk and egg white. Heat a non-stick pan on medium-low heat. Slowly melt 1 teaspoon of the butter in the pan. If the butter sizzles and pops, the pan is too hot. Add the eggs to the pan and season with salt and pepper. Stir the eggs and shake the pan to make sure that no eggs are sticking to the pan. Loosen around the edges with a spatula while the eggs cook. After 20 seconds of cooking, remove pan from the heat. Allow the omelet to sit off the heat for 1 minute. Fold the omelet in thirds and serve. Top with remaining butter, chives, and cheese.

Nutritional Information (per omelet):
Calories: 321.6
Fat: 27.2 g
Cholesterol: 422.5 mg
Sodium: 803.1 mg
Potassium: 144.9 mg
Carbohydrate: 0.9 mg
Protein: 19.7 g

Scrambled Eggs with Ham

Prep Time: 5 minutes
Cook Time: 10 minutes
Yield: 4 servings

Ingredients:
8 oz. cured ham steak
1 T. extra virgin olive oil
8 eggs, beaten
3 T. heavy cream
1/4 tsp. kosher salt
1/4 tsp. freshly ground pepper
2 T. parsley leaves, minced

Directions:
Sear ham steak in a skillet over medium heat until browned and hot throughout. Remove from the skillet and dice into ½" cubes. Set aside. In a medium bowl, mix eggs, cream, salt, and pepper. Heat olive oil in the skillet until shimmering. Pour in egg mixture and stir until large lumps of cooked egg have formed (about 2 minutes). Continue cooking, stirring gently, until no uncooked egg remains. Remove from heat and stir in ham cubes. Serve warm garnished with parsley.

Nutritional Information (per serving):
Calories: 262.9
Fat: 17.3 g
Cholesterol: 412.9 mg
Sodium: 986.9 mg
Potassium: 342.9 mg
Carbohydrate: 1.3 g
Protein: 24.0 g

Fiesta Sausage and Egg Open-Faced Sandwich

Prep Time: 5 minutes
Cook Time: 10 minutes
Yield: 2 sandwiches

Ingredients:
1 vanilla almond waffle, quartered (pg. 47)
4 eggs
4 pork sausage patties
4 slices sharp cheddar cheese
1/2 c. prepared salsa
1 T. unsalted butter
1/2 tsp. kosher salt
1/4 tsp. freshly ground black pepper

Directions:
Brown sausage patties in a skillet over medium-high heat. Set aside. Heat butter in the skillet until melted and bubbling. Fry eggs until desired doneness, seasoning with salt and pepper. Top each waffle quarter with a sausage patty, a fried egg, a slice of cheese, and 2 tablespoons salsa.

Nutritional Information (per sandwich):
Calories: 543.7
Fat: 39.7 g
Cholesterol: 214.0 mg
Sodium: 879.1 mg
Potassium: 604.8 mg
Carbohydrate: 11.7 g
Protein: 24.1 g

Spinach Bacon Frittata
Prep Time: 5 minutes
Cook Time: 20 minutes
Yield: 4 servings

Ingredients:
4 slices thick-cut bacon
1 medium onion, halved and sliced
1 clove garlic, minced
1 (10 oz.) package frozen spinach, thawed
6 eggs, beaten
1/4 tsp. kosher salt
1/4 tsp. freshly ground black pepper

Directions:
Preheat oven to 400°F. Cook bacon in a cast-iron (or other oven-safe) skillet over medium heat until crisp. Set aside. Sauté onions and garlic in the bacon grease for 5 minutes. Squeeze excess liquid from the spinach and add to the pan. Crumble bacon and distribute evenly among the spinach mixture. Pour in eggs and season with salt and pepper. Cook the frittata on the stove for 2 minutes, scraping around the edges with a spatula. Finish baking in the oven until the top is set, 10-12 minutes. Serve warm or cool.

Nutritional Information (per serving):
Calories: 205.3
Fat: 12.9 g
Cholesterol: 291.5 mg
Sodium: 453.7 mg
Potassium: 315.2 mg
Carbohydrate: 6.3 g
Protein: 15.6 g

Coconut Zucchini Muffins

Prep Time: 10 minutes
Cook Time: 25 minutes
Yield: 12 muffins

Ingredients:
2/3 c. coconut flour
1 tsp. baking soda
1/2 tsp. kosher salt
4 grams stevia powder*
1/2 tsp. ground cinnamon
1/4 c. coconut oil, melted
4 eggs, beaten
1/4 c. plain yogurt
1 c. shredded zucchini
1/2 c. shredded unsweetened coconut

Directions:
Preheat oven to 350°F. In a large bowl, combine flour, soda, stevia powder, salt, and cinnamon. Set aside. In a medium bowl, mix coconut oil, eggs, and yogurt until well combined. Pour the egg mixture into the flour mixture and stir until just incorporated. Add the zucchini and coconut. Scoop into greased or lined muffin tins and bake for 20-25 minutes.

*This recipe can be sweetened with any low- or no-carb sweetener of your choice.

Nutritional Information (per muffin):
Calories: 114.4
Fat: 9.8 g
Cholesterol: 63.3 mg
Sodium: 214.8 mg

Potassium: 77.3 mg
Carbohydrate: 3.8 g
Protein: 3.9 g

Vanilla Almond Waffle

Prep Time: 10 minutes
Cook Time: 15 minutes
Yield: 6 servings

Ingredients:
1/2 c. almond flour
1/4 c. vanilla protein powder
1/4 tsp. baking soda
1 tsp. baking powder
1/2 tsp. kosher salt
2 grams stevia powder (or sweetener of choice)
4 eggs, separated
1/2 c. unsweetened vanilla almond milk
2 T. coconut oil, melted
1/2 c. heavy cream, whipped
1 c. fresh raspberries

Directions:
After separating, put egg whites in a medium metal bowl in the refrigerator to chill. In a large bowl, combine the almond flour, protein powder, soda, baking powder, salt, and sweetener. Set aside. In another bowl, whisk together egg yolks, almond milk, and coconut oil. Pour liquid mixture into the almond flour bowl and stir to combine.

Remove egg whites from the refrigerator and beat to stiff peaks with a handheld electric mixer. Gently stir 1/3 of the egg white mixture into the batter. Gently fold in the remaining egg whites. Pour batter into a greased waffle maker and cook until golden brown and slightly crisp on the outside. Serve with whipped cream and raspberries. Alternate toppings could include blueberries and unsweetened coconut, shredded cheese and green onions, or sugar-free caramel flavoring syrup with toasted almonds.

Nutritional Information (per waffle):
Calories: 250.1
Fat: 20.0 g
Cholesterol: 156.2 mg
Sodium: 411.1 mg
Potassium: 116.6 mg
Carbohydrate: 5.6 g
Protein: 14.1 g

Lox and Cream Cheese Boats
Prep Time: 5 minutes
Yield: 2 servings

Ingredients:
8 oz. smoked salmon, thinly sliced
1 (3 oz.) package cream cheese, softened
1 cucumber, peeled
2 tsp. extra virgin olive oil
1/2 tsp. kosher salt

Directions:
Slice cucumber in half and scoop out seeds. Slice each section in half again, resulting in four cucumber "boats." Spread cream cheese in the empty seed cavity of each cucumber section. Layer 2 oz. salmon on each cucumber. Top with a drizzle of olive oil and salt to taste.

Nutritional Information (per serving):
Calories: 329.8
Fat: 24.4 g
Cholesterol: 72.6 mg
Sodium: 288 g
Potassium: 393.6 mg
Carbohydrate: 3.9 g
Protein: 24.5 g

Nut and Seed Breakfast Biscuits

Prep Time: 10 minutes
Cook Time: 15 minutes
Yield: 2-dozen biscuits

Ingredients:
2 1/4 c. almond flour
1/2 tsp. baking soda
1/2 tsp. baking powder
1 tsp. kosher salt
1/2 c. sunflower seeds
1/2 c. pecans, chopped
1/2 c. walnuts, chopped
4 T. unsalted butter, melted
4 T. coconut oil, melted
2 tsp. stevia powder
1 egg, beaten
2 tsp. vanilla extract

Directions:
Preheat oven to 350°F. Mix flour, soda, powder, salt, seeds, and nuts in a medium bowl. Set aside. In another bowl, combine butter, coconut oil, maple syrup, egg, and vanilla. Stir until well-mixed. Pour butter mixture into the dry ingredients. Mix until just combined.

Scoop 1 tablespoon at a time onto a parchment-lined baking sheet. Bake for 15 minutes. Cool on the baking sheet for extra crispy biscuits.

Nutritional Information (per 2 cookies):
Calories: 299.1
Fat: 28.8 g

Cholesterol: 25.9 mg
Sodium: 239.5 mg
Potassium: 95.8 mg
Carbohydrate: 7.3 g
Protein: 7.3 g

Baked Vanilla Custard

Prep Time: 15 minutes
Cook Time: 1 hour
Yield: 6 servings

Ingredients:
1 c. heavy cream
1 c. unsweetened almond milk
2 eggs
3 egg yolks
1 T. granulated sugar
1 T. vanilla extract
1/2 tsp. ground nutmeg

Directions:
Preheat oven to 325°F. Place a shallow pan of hot water on the bottom rack of the oven while it preheats. This will provide the humidity needed to bake the custard properly. Scald cream and almond milk over medium heat. Do not boil. When the cream mixture is steaming, remove from heat.

Whisk eggs, sugar, and vanilla extract in a large bowl. Drizzle in 1/2 c. of the hot cream mixture while continuing to whisk. Once the eggs are hot, stir in the remainder of the cream mixture. Pour mixture through a fine-mesh strainer into a shallow pie or casserole dish. Top with nutmeg and bake 1 hour. Serve warm.

Nutritional Information (per serving):
Calories: 208.4
Fat: 19.0 g
Cholesterol: 208.3 mg
Sodium: 68.0 mg
Potassium: 92.2 mg

Carbohydrate: 4.2 g
Protein: 4.4 g

Overnight Chia Pudding

Prep Time: 5 minutes
Chill Time: 6+ hours
Yield: 6 servings

Ingredients:
2 c. unsweetened vanilla almond milk
1/2 c. chia seeds

Directions:
Combine milk and seeds in a medium bowl or container with a lid. Cover and chill overnight. Stir before serving. Garnish with fresh berries, chopped nuts, or a drizzle of honey.

Nutritional Information (per serving):
Calories: 90.0
Fat: 4.8 g
Cholesterol: 0.0 mg
Sodium: 50.0 mg
Potassium: 133.3 mg
Total Carbohydrate: 7.0 g
*Net Carbohydrate: 0.0 g
Protein: 4.3 g

Warm Flax Cereal

Prep Time: 5 minutes
Cook Time: 3 minutes
Yield: 3 servings

Ingredients:
1 T. unsalted butter
1/2 c. flax seed meal
2/3 c. hot water
2 T. full-fat buttermilk
1/2 tsp. cinnamon
1/4 tsp. ground nutmeg

Directions:
Melt butter in a medium saucepan. Remove from heat and add flax seed meal, stirring to combine. Mix hot water with the flax seed mixture and let sit for 3 minutes. Serve with buttermilk, cinnamon, and nutmeg.

Nutritional Information (per serving):
Calories: 149.2
Fat: 10.1 g
Cholesterol: 14.0 mg
Sodium: 27.5 mg
Potassium: 79.8 mg
Total Carbohydrate: 8.3 g
*Net Carbohydrate: 2.7 g
Protein: 5.8 g

Drinks and Smoothies
Bulletproof Coffee
Prep Time: 5 minutes
Yield: 2 servings

Ingredients:
2 c. brewed coffee
2 T. unsalted butter (from grass-fed cows is best), melted
1 T. coconut oil, melted

Directions:
Blend all ingredients with an immersion blender for 10-15 seconds until frothy. Flavor variations include vanilla latte (add 1 tablespoon heavy cream and 1 tsp. vanilla extract), spiced Turkish-style (add 1/4 teaspoon each of cinnamon and ground cardamom), or chocolate cream (add 1/2 teaspoon cocoa powder and 1 tablespoon heavy cream). For a higher fat content, substitute 1 tablespoon MCT oil for the coconut oil.

Nutritional Information (per serving):
Calories: 162.4
Fat: 18.3 g
Cholesterol: 31.1 mg
Sodium: 6.6 mg
Potassium: 119.9 mg
Carbohydrate: 0.0 g
Protein: 0.4 g

Cinnamon Almond Milk

Prep Time: 5 minutes
Yield: 2 servings

Ingredients:
2 c. unsweetened vanilla almond milk
1/2 c. heavy cream
1 tsp. ground cinnamon
1/8 tsp. ground nutmeg

Directions:
Combine almond milk and cream in a large measuring cup or blender. Blending the milk and cream will produce a frothier drink. Garnish with cinnamon and nutmeg. Serve warm or cold.

Nutritional Information (per serving):
Calories: 239.0
Fat: 24.6 g
Cholesterol: 81.5 mg
Sodium: 172.9 mg
Potassium: 210.8 mg
Carbohydrate: 3.6 g
Protein: 2.3 g

Strawberries and Cream Smoothie

Prep Time: 5 minutes
Yield: 1 serving

Ingredients:
1 c. unsweetened vanilla almond milk
1/4 c. frozen strawberries
1 oz. cream cheese, softened
1 scoop vanilla protein powder

Directions:
Blend all ingredients until smooth. For a thicker smoothie, freeze half of the almond milk in ice cube trays before using. Xantham gum can also be added for a thicker consistency.

Nutritional Information (per serving):
Calories: 240.0
Fat: 12.3 g
Cholesterol: 46.0 mg
Sodium: 384.6 mg
Potassium: 334.1 mg
Carbohydrate: 8.6 g
Protein: 25.3 g

Iced Green Tea
Prep Time: 5 minutes
Yield: 1 serving

Ingredients:
1 c. unsweetened vanilla almond milk
1 scoop vanilla protein powder
1 tsp. green tea powder
1 gram stevia powder

Directions:
Blend all ingredients until smooth. Serve over ice. For something closer to a smoothie, blend in 1/2 cup ice with the other ingredients.

Nutritional Information:
Calories: 146.0
Fat: 2.5 g
Cholesterol 15.0 mg
Sodium: 300.0 mg
Potassium: 240.2 mg
Carbohydrate: 4.5 g
Protein: 23.0 g

Pumpkin Spice Smoothie

Prep Time: 5 minutes
Yield: 1 serving

Ingredients:
1 c. unsweetened vanilla almond milk
2 T. pumpkin puree
1 scoop vanilla protein powder
2 grams stevia powder
1/2 tsp. cinnamon
1/8 tsp. ground ginger
1/8 tsp. ground nutmeg
1/8 tsp. ground cloves
2 T. heavy cream, whipped
1 tsp. sugar-free caramel syrup

Directions:
Blend all ingredients until smooth. This smoothie can also be served warm. Xantham gum can also be added for a thicker consistency.

Nutritional Information:
Calories: 249.6
Fat: 13.9 g
Cholesterol: 56.1 mg
Sodium: 314.1 mg
Potassium: 275.1 mg
*Net Carbohydrate: 5.0 g
Protein: 24.2 g

Chocolate Peanut Butter Smoothie

Prep Time: 5 minutes
Yield: 2 servings

Ingredients:
1/2 avocado
1/4 c. natural peanut butter
1 T. unsweetened cocoa powder
2 grams stevia powder
1/2 c. unsweetened coconut milk

Directions:
Blend all ingredients until smooth. For a thicker smoothie, freeze half of the coconut milk in ice cube trays before using. Xantham gum can also be added for a thicker consistency.

Nutritional Information (per serving):
Calories: 296.2
Fat: 23.6 g
Cholesterol: 0.0 mg
Sodium: 160.6 mg
Potassium: 231.1 mg
*Net Carbohydrate: 5.6 g
Protein: 9.0 g

Thick and Creamy Vanilla Shake
Prep Time: 5 minutes
Yield: 1 serving

Ingredients:
4-6 ice cubes
1 c. unsweetened vanilla almond milk
1 scoop vanilla protein powder
1/4 c. heavy cream
1 oz. sugar-free vanilla flavoring
1/4 tsp. xantham gum

Directions:
Blend all ingredients until smooth. For a thicker smoothie, freeze half of the coconut milk in ice cube trays before using. Other flavors of sugar-free syrup can be used to make creamy shakes in other flavor combinations such as strawberry, chocolate, turtle (chocolate and caramel), Neapolitan (three 1/3 batches in strawberry, chocolate, and vanilla layered in the glass), or chocolate-dipped strawberry (chocolate and strawberry).

Nutritional Information (per serving):
Calories: 338.7
Fat: 24.5 g
Cholesterol: 96.5 mg
Sodium: 327.6 mg
Potassium: 284.6 mg
Carbohydrate: 5.7 g
Protein: 24.2 g

Soups and Stews

Bacon and Cheese Broccoli Soup

Prep Time: 5 minutes
Cook Time: 20 minutes
Yield: 8 servings

Ingredients:
4 slices thick-cut bacon
2 cloves garlic, minced
1 medium onion, diced
4 c. chicken stock
2 heads broccoli, chopped
1 c. frozen spinach, thawed
1 (4 oz.) package cream cheese, cubed
1/2 c. heavy cream
1 c. shredded sharp cheddar cheese
kosher salt

Directions:
In a large, heavy-bottomed pot, cook bacon until crisp. Set aside. Sauté onion and garlic in the rendered bacon fat until the onions are translucent. Add stock and broccoli. Bring to a boil, then reduce heat to maintain a low boil. Cook for 10 minutes or until broccoli is tender. Reduce heat to low and add spinach. Use an immersion blender to puree the soup until smooth. Stir in cream cheese and cheddar cheese one handful at a time, letting the cheese melt completely before adding more. When the cheese is fully incorporated, add salt to taste. Serve garnished with chopped bacon.

Nutritional Information (per serving):
Calories: 276.1
Fat: 18.9 g

Cholesterol: 58.2 mg
Sodium: 491.5 mg
Carbohydrate: 9.7 g
Protein: 14.6 g

Lemon Rosemary Chicken Soup
Prep Time: 10 minutes
Cook Time: 20 minutes
Yield: 6 servings

Ingredients:
2 T. extra virgin olive oil
1 lb. boneless, skinless chicken thighs, cubed
3 cloves garlic, minced
1 medium onion, diced
3 carrots, diced
2 stalks celery, diced
1 T. fresh thyme leaves
2 bay leaves
1 sprig rosemary
4 c. chicken stock
zest and juice of 1 lemon
kosher salt

Directions:
Heat oil in a large stock pot until simmering. Add chicken to the pot and cook until browned. Add garlic, onion, carrots, and celery. Cook for 4-5 minutes or until the onions are translucent, stirring occasionally to keep the garlic from scorching. Add herbs and chicken stock. Bring to a boil, then reduce to maintain a steady simmer. Simmer 15 minutes. Stir in lemon zest and juice. Salt to taste and serve.

Nutritional Information (per serving):
Calories 131.5
Fat: 6.8 g
Cholesterol: 10.5 mg

Sodium: 435.1 mg
Potassium: 381.9 mg
Carbohydrate: 11.8 g
Protein: 6.1 g

White Chicken Crockpot Chili

Prep Time: 5 minutes
Cook Time: 6+ hours
Yield: 6 servings

Ingredients:
1 T. canola oil
1/2 c. diced onion
2 cloves garlic, minced
1 jalapeño, diced
1 1/2 lb. boneless, skinless chicken thighs
1 (28 oz.) can diced tomatoes
4 c. chicken stock
2 tsp. ground cumin
1 tsp. kosher salt
1/2 tsp. freshly ground pepper
1 tsp. dried oregano
1 T. chili powder
3 oz. cream cheese, cubed
1/2 c. heavy cream

Garnishes:
sour cream
cheddar cheese
cilantro, chopped
avocado

Directions:
In a large skillet, heat oil until shimmering. Cook onion, garlic, and jalapeño for 2-3 minutes or until fragrant. Scrape onion mixture into the bowl of a 5-quart crockpot. Add the chicken, tomatoes, chicken stock, cumin, salt, pepper, oregano, and chili

powder. Cook on low for 6-8 hours. Remove chicken and shred into bite-sized pieces. Return chicken to the pot and add cream cheese and heavy cream, stirring until the cream cheese is fully incorporated. Serve immediately with desired garnishes.

Nutritional Information (per serving):
Calories: 248.1
Fat: 17.1 g
Cholesterol: 56.0 mg
Sodium: 912.0 mg
Potassium: 282.2 mg
Carbohydrate: 10.2 g
Protein: 9.1 g

Chicken Sausage and Kale Soup

Prep Time: 10 minutes
Cook Time: 30 minutes
Yield: 6 servings

Ingredients:
2 slices thick-cut bacon
1 lb. Andouille sausage, sliced 1/4" thick
2 c. button mushrooms, sliced
6 cloves garlic, minced
3 c. kale, washed and chopped
1 tsp. kosher salt
1/2 tsp. black pepper
4 c. chicken stock
2 T. red wine vinegar

Directions:
Cook bacon in a large soup pot over medium-high heat until crisp. Set aside. (Another option is to bake the bacon on a foil-lined, rimmed baking sheet for 15-20 minutes at 425°F. In this case, reserve 2 tablespoons fat from the baking sheet for browning the sausage.) Brown the sausage in the rendered bacon fat and set aside. Sauté the kale, mushrooms, and garlic in the pot for 2-3 minutes or until the kale has started to wilt and the garlic is fragrant. Season with salt and pepper. Add chicken stock and simmer for 20 minutes. Return sausage to the pot and cook until heated through. Serve with a splash of red wine vinegar and crumbled bacon.

Nutritional Information (per serving):
Calories: 218.0
Fat: 11.4 g

Cholesterol: 42.3 mg
Sodium: 1.03 g
Potassium: 330.4 mg
Carbohydrate: 6.7 g
Protein: 17.5 g

Curried Shrimp Soup
Prep Time: 10 minutes
Cook Time: 40 minutes
Yield: 6 servings

Ingredients:
1 T. unsalted butter
3 cloves garlic, minced
1 jalapeño, diced
1 medium onion, diced
1 T. fresh ginger, grated
2 T. red curry paste
1 (12 oz.) can diced tomatoes
1 (13 oz.) can unsweetened coconut milk
4 c. chicken stock
2 lb. raw shrimp, peeled and deveined
kosher salt
freshly ground black pepper
1/4 c. fresh cilantro, chopped
1 lime, quartered

Directions:
Melt butter in a large soup pot over medium heat until bubbling. Add garlic, jalapeño, onion, ginger, and sauté 2-3 minutes or until the onions are translucent but not browned. Add curry paste and cook until fragrant (3 minutes more). Mix in tomatoes, coconut milk, and chicken stock. Simmer for 15 minutes. Add shrimp and cook until the shrimp is cooked through (5-7 minutes). Season to taste. Serve with cilantro and lime as garnishes.

Nutritional Information (per serving):

Calories: 335.0
Fat: 17.0 g
Cholesterol: 238.2 mg
Sodium: 1.35 g
Potassium: 625.5 mg
Carbohydrate: 10.7 g
Protein: 33.0 g

Main Dishes

Tandoori-Style Grilled Chicken

Prep Time: 4+ hours
Cook Time: 30 minutes
Yield: 6 servings

Ingredients:
4 lb. chicken breast with skin
1 c. whole milk plain yogurt
6 cloves garlic, minced
2 T. fresh ginger, grated
1/4 c. lemon juice
2 tsp. kosher salt
1 T. ground cumin
1 T. smoked paprika
1 T. ground coriander
1 1/2 tsp. turmeric
1/2 tsp. ground cloves
1/2 tsp. ground cardamom

Directions:
Combine yogurt, garlic, ginger, lemon juice, and salt in a large bowl. Mix in the remaining spices until combined. Submerge the chicken quarters in the yogurt-spice mixture and cover. Marinate in the refrigerator at least 4 hours and up to overnight.

An hour before serving, preheat an outdoor grill or grill pan to medium-high heat. When the grill is hot, remove chicken from the marinade and wipe excess yogurt from the chicken. Char chicken 7 minutes per side, then reduce the heat to medium-low. Cook, covered, an additional 15 minutes or the interior of the chicken reaches 165°F. Let rest, tented with foil, for 15 minutes before serving.

Nutritional Information (per serving):
Calories: 143.0
Fat: 7.2 g
Cholesterol: 42.4 mg
Sodium: 697.6 mg
Potassium: 264.9 mg
Carbohydrate: 5.9 g
Protein: 14.1 g

Trout en Papillote with Olive Tapenade
Prep Time: 10 minutes
Cook Time: 10 minutes
Yield: 4 servings

Ingredients:
1 c. pitted mixed olives
1 anchovy fillet, rinsed
1 clove garlic, minced
1 T. capers
1/4 c. fresh parsley leaves
4 trout fillets
2 lemons, sliced
white wine
extra virgin olive oil
kosher salt
freshly ground black pepper

Directions:
Preheat oven to 400°F. Prepare the tapenade by combining the first 5 ingredients in a food processor 1-2 minutes. Add a drizzle of olive oil if the texture is too thick. Set aside.

Lay each fillet on a piece of parchment paper about 15 inches square. Top each fillet with 3 lemon slices. Season with salt and pepper. Drizzle with oil and a splash of white wine each. Fold edges of the paper to form a packet around the fish. Place on a baking sheet and bake until the fish flakes easily with a fork (about 10 minutes).

Nutritional Information (per serving):
Calories: 315.5

Fat: 17.1 g
Cholesterol: 99.5 mg
Sodium: 530.7 mg
Potassium: 755.6 mg
Carbohydrate: 8.5 g
Protein: 33.9 g

Salmon Cakes
Prep Time: 20 minutes
Cook Time: 15 minutes
Yield: 4 servings

Ingredients:
1 (15 oz.) can pink salmon
1/4 c. crushed pork rinds
1/2 c. chopped onion
1.4 c. parsley leaves, chopped
2 eggs, beaten
3 T. canola oil

Directions:
Empty salmon into a large bowl and shred with a fork. Stir in pork rinds, onion, parsley, and eggs. Form into 4 equally-sized patties and chill for 15 minutes. While the salmon cakes are chilling, heat oil in a large cast iron skillet or griddle. Pan fry cakes for 5-7 minutes per side, or until golden brown. Serve with fresh lemon juice.

Nutritional Information (per serving):
Calories: 414.5
Fat: 25.9 g
Cholesterol: 191.4 mg
Sodium: 657.9 mg
Carbohydrate: 2.2 g
Protein: 42.5 g

Curried Egg Salad
Prep Time: 2+ hours
Cook Time: 12 minutes
Yield: 4 servings

Ingredients:
12 eggs
1/2 c. mayonnaise
1/2 c. celery, diced
1 medium dill pickle, diced
1 tsp. curry powder
1/4 c. smoked paprika
1/2 tsp. kosher salt
1/4 tsp. freshly ground pepper

Directions:
Place eggs in a large pot with a lid and cover with cold water. Cook, uncovered, on medium-high heat until boiling. Once the water boils, remove from heat and cover. Let the eggs sit for 12 minutes. Drain immediately and rinse in cold water. Peel the eggs when cool enough to handle. Finely chop eggs once peeled.

While the eggs cook, combine mayonnaise, pickle, celery, curry powder, paprika, salt, and pepper. Add eggs to the mayonnaise mixture and chill at least 2 hours before serving.

Nutritional Information (per serving):
Calories: 421.5
Fat: 36.0 g
Cholesterol: 565.6 mg
Sodium: 787.6 mg
Potassium: 265.9 mg

Carbohydrate: 3.5 g
Protein: 19.4 g

Pork and Green Bean Stir Fry with Peanut Sauce
Prep Time: 30 minutes
Cook Time: 15 minutes
Yield: 4 servings

Ingredients:
1 lb. pork tenderloin, sliced into thin strips
3 T. soy sauce, divided
2 cloves garlic, minced
1/4 tsp. crushed red pepper flakes
3 T. natural peanut butter
1 tsp. sesame oil
1 T. rice wine vinegar
2 c. green beans, trimmed
1 T. canola oil
1/4 c. dry-roasted peanuts

Directions:
Mix pork, 2 tablespoons soy sauce, garlic, and red pepper flakes in a medium bowl and marinade 15-30 minutes. In another bowl, whisk together peanut butter, sesame oil, vinegar, and 1 tablespoon soy sauce. Cover green beans with water in a large skillet and boil until green beans are almost tender (about 3 minutes). Strain green beans and return the skillet to medium-high heat. Heat oil until shimmering, then add the pork mixture. Stir fry 5-7 minutes or until the pork is cooked through. Return green beans to the skillet and add the peanut butter mixture. Cook until heated through, about 2 minutes. Garnish with peanuts and serve.

Nutritional Information (per serving):
Calories: 426.6

Fat: 24.5 g
Cholesterol: 89.6 mg
Sodium: 788.1 mg
Potassium: 582.9 mg
Carbohydrate: 9.6 g
Protein: 40.3 g

Garlic and Lemon Roast Chicken
Prep Time: 5 minutes
Cook Time: 1 hour
Yield: 6 servings

Ingredients:
1 whole chicken, in pieces
4 lemons, sliced
10 cloves of garlic, peeled
2 T. extra virgin olive oil
1 tsp. kosher salt
1/4 tsp. freshly ground black pepper

Directions:
Preheat oven to 350°F. Arrange chicken pieces in a large roasting pan and rub with olive oil. Season liberally with salt and pepper. Arrange lemon slices and garlic cloves around the chicken. Bake for 1 hour. Let rest, covered, 10 minutes before serving.

Nutritional Information (per serving):
Calories: 418.7
Fat: 26.2 g
Cholesterol: 98.3 mg
Sodium: 323.0 mg
Potassium: 125.6 mg
Carbohydrate: 9.4 g
Protein: 38.5 g

Chicken Piccata

Prep Time: 15 minutes
Cook Time: 20 minutes
Yield: 4 servings

Ingredients:
2 boneless, skinless chicken breasts
2/3 c. crushed pork rinds
6 T. butter
5 T. extra virgin olive oil
1/3 c. lemon juice
1/2 c. chicken stock
1/4 c. capers
kosher salt
freshly ground pepper

Directions:
Butterfly chicken breasts, then slice in half. You will be left with 4 chicken cutlets. Season chicken with salt and pepper, then dredge in pork rinds. Melt 2 tablespoons butter with 3 tablespoons olive oil over medium heat. Add 2 pieces of chicken and cook for 3 minutes per side. Set aside. Melt an additional 2 tablespoons butter with 2 tablespoons olive oil and repeat with the remaining chicken.

Once the final chicken cutlets have been browned and set aside, turn the heat to medium-high. Deglaze the pan with the lemon juice, stock, and capers by stirring constantly to scrape up any bits stuck to the pan. Reduce the heat to maintain a simmer and check for seasoning. Add additional salt and pepper if desired. Return the chicken to the pan with the remaining 2 tablespoons butter and simmer for 5 minutes before serving.

Nutritional Information (per serving):
Calories: 533.1
Fat: 42.9 g
Cholesterol: 135.3 mg
Sodium: 771.5 mg
Potassium: 307.9 mg
Carbohydrate: 3.2 g
Protein: 36.6 g

Chicken Salad with Avocado

Prep Time: 10 minutes
Yield: 4 servings

Ingredients:
2 c. shredded chicken
1/2 c. chopped celery
1/2 tsp. kosher salt
1/4 tsp. freshly ground black pepper
1/4 tsp. garlic powder
1 T. lime juice
3 T. cream cheese, softened
1 avocado, smashed

Directions:
Combine all ingredients in a large bowl and mix until the cream cheese and avocado are completely incorporated. Add more lime juice to taste.

Nutritional Information (per serving):
Calories: 250.0
Fat: 13.5 g
Cholesterol: 82.1 mg
Sodium: 349.4 mg
Potassium: 493.1 mg
Carbohydrate: 4.9 g
Protein: 27.5 g

Crunchy Low-Carb Chicken Strips

Prep Time: 15 minutes
Cook Time: 10 minutes
Yield: 4 servings

Ingredients:
3 c. pork rinds, crushed
1 tsp. garlic powder
1 lb. chicken tenders
2 eggs, beaten
1/2 c. Parmesan cheese, grated
4 T. coconut oil

Directions:
Crush pork rinds and mix with garlic powder and cheese in a shallow bowl or pie dish. Heat oil in a cast-iron skillet over medium-high heat. Dip chicken tenders in egg then in pork rind mixture, turning to coat. Pan fry tenders in the hot oil until golden brown, turning once (about 5 minutes per side).

Nutritional Information (per serving):
Calories: 442.6
Fat: 28.3 g
Cholesterol: 197.9 mg
Sodium: 718.4 mg
Potassium: 55.6 mg
Carbohydrate: 1.2 g
Protein: 47.0 g

Steak with Chimichurri Sauce

Prep Time: 10 minutes
Cook Time: 30 minutes
Yield: 4 servings

Ingredients:
1 c. packed Italian parsley leaves
1 c. packed cilantro leaves
4 cloves garlic, peeled
4 tsp. dried oregano
1 shallot, peeled and sliced in half
1 jalapeño, seeded
1/4 c. red wine vinegar
1/2 tsp. kosher salt
3/4 c. extra virgin olive oil
2 New York strip steaks
2 T. canola oil
kosher salt
freshly ground black pepper

Directions:
For the sauce (can be done ahead): Pulse parsley, cilantro, garlic, oregano, shallot, jalapeño, and vinegar in the bowl of a food processor until finely minced. Add salt. Slowly drizzle in olive oil while continuing to pulse the mixture. Refrigerate the chimichurri until ready to serve.

For the steak:
Preheat grill to high. Brush steaks with oil and season with salt and pepper. Sear steaks on grill and cook for 5 minutes. Flip once and cook for 5-10 minutes more, depending on desired doneness. Transfer the steaks to a cutting board and tent with

foil. Allow to rest for 15 minutes. Slice steaks and serve with chimichurri sauce.

Nutritional Information (per serving):

Calories: 613.5

Fat: 56.3 g

Cholesterol: 49.0 mg

Sodium: 419.8 mg

Potassium: 36.9 mg

Carbohydrate: 3.9 g

Protein: 26.0 g

Chicken Liver and Onions

Prep Time: 5 minutes
Cook Time: 18 minutes
Yield: 4 servings

Ingredients:
1 lb. chicken livers
2 medium onions, sliced
4 T. unsalted butter
1/2 tsp. kosher salt
1 tsp. garlic powder

Directions:
Heat butter in a large skillet over medium heat. Season livers with salt and garlic powder. Once the butter is melted and bubbling, add livers and onions to the skillet. Cook until the onions are translucent and the livers cooked through (about 15 minutes).

Nutritional Information (per serving):
Calories: 128.0
Fat: 11.7 g
Cholesterol: 39.7 mg
Sodium: 245.2 mg
Potassium: 103.5 mg
Carbohydrate: 5.3 g
Protein: 1.3 g

Slow Cooker Pot Roast

Prep Time: 5 minutes
Cook Time: 6-8 hours
Yield: 8 servings

Ingredients:
4 lb. chuck roast
2 c. mushrooms, sliced
4 carrots, peeled
2 medium onions, quartered
6 cloves garlic, peeled
2 tsp. kosher salt
freshly ground black pepper
1 bay leaf
1/4 c. water

Directions:
Place roast at the bottom of the bowl of a 5-quart crock pot. Layer mushrooms, carrots, and onions on top of the roast. Tuck garlic around the edges and season with salt, pepper, and bay leaf. Add water and cover. Cook on low for 6-8 hours or until the roast falls apart.

Nutritional Information (per serving):
Calories: 437.1
Fat: 31.1 g
Cholesterol: 116.0 mg
Sodium: 574.9 mg
Potassium: 205.2 mg
Carbohydrate: 6.6 g
Protein: 33.3 g

Glazed Bacon Meatloaf

Prep Time: 5 minutes
Cook Time: 1 hour
Yield: 8 servings

Ingredients:
1 lb. ground beef
1 lb. ground pork
2 eggs, beaten
1 c. Parmesan cheese, grated
1/2 tsp. kosher salt
1/4 tsp. freshly ground black pepper
1 T. Worcestershire sauce
8 slices thick-cut bacon
1/2 c. reduced-sugar ketchup
1 T. apricot preserves
1 tsp. mustard

Directions:
Preheat oven to 350°F. Combine beef, pork, eggs, cheese, salt, pepper, and Worcestershire sauce in a large mixing bowl. Form the mixture into a loaf shape on a broiler pan and top with bacon, tucking the ends of the bacon under the loaf if they hang over the sides. In a separate bowl, combine ketchup, apricot preserves, and mustard. Spread half the ketchup mixture over the top of the meatloaf. Bake for 55 minutes, adding the remainder of the glaze 30 minutes through cooking time.

Nutritional Information (per serving):
Calories: 482.8
Fat: 36.3 g
Cholesterol: 162.8 mg

Sodium: 820.7 mg
Potassium: 366.8 mg
Carbohydrate: 3.7 g
Protein: 32.8 g

Spaghetti Squash with Meaty Marinara
Prep Time: 5 minutes
Cook Time: 45 minutes
Yield: 4 servings

Ingredients:
1 large spaghetti squash
1 medium onion, diced
2 cloves garlic, minced
1 lb. ground beef
1 bay leaf
1 tsp. dried basil
1/2 tsp. dried oregano
1/2 tsp. red pepper flakes
1 (28-oz.) can whole, peeled tomatoes
1 T. capers
1 T. red wine vinegar
kosher salt

Directions:
Preheat oven to 400°F. Slice spaghetti squash lengthwise and discard the seeds. For longer strands of squash, slice the squash into 2" rounds instead of slicing lengthwise. Place squash with the cut side up in a shallow roasting pan and sprinkle with salt. Roast for 30 minutes. Allow the squash to cool slightly before removing the skin and separating the squash into thin noodles with a fork.

While the squash roasts, prepare the sauce. Heat oil in a stockpot over medium heat. Add the onion and cook until translucent but not browned. Add the garlic and cook, stirring constantly, for 30 seconds. Add the ground beef and cook until browned, breaking apart chunks with a spatula or spoon. When the beef is cooked through, add the spices and tomatoes. Bring the mixture to a boil, then reduce the heat to maintain a low simmer for at least 30 minutes. Prior to serving, remove the bay leaf and add capers and vinegar. Season with salt to taste.

Nutritional Information (per serving):
Calories: 311.1
Fat: 21.4 g
Cholesterol: 70.0 mg
Sodium: 398.3 mg
Potassium: 244.8 mg
Carbohydrate: 9.6 g
Protein: 21.4 g

Vegetables and Sides
Cauliflower "Rice"
Prep Time: 5 minutes
Cook Time: 10 minutes
Yield: 4 servings

Ingredients:
1 large head cauliflower, trimmed
2 T. extra virgin olive oil
1/2 c. chopped shallots
1 tsp. kosher salt

Directions:
Pulse cauliflower florets in a food processor in batches until broken down to the size of rice or couscous. Avoid processing the tough stems or leaves. Heat oil in a large pot or saucepan over medium heat. Add the cauliflower and onions, stirring frequently for 2 minutes. Stir in salt and cover for an additional 2-4 minutes or until cauliflower is soft.

Nutritional Information (per serving):
Calories: 119.7
Fat: 7.5 g
Cholesterol: 0.0 g
Sodium: 544.2 mg
Potassium: 669.7 mg
Carbohydrate: 12.6 g
*Net Carbohydrate: 9.0 g
Protein: 4.4 g

Caprese Salad
Prep Time: 5 minutes
Yield: 4 servings

Ingredients:
2 fresh tomatoes, sliced
9 oz. fresh mozzarella, sliced
12 basil leaves, stems removed
3 T. balsamic vinegar
3 T. extra virgin olive oil
1/2 tsp. kosher salt

Directions:
Whisk together vinegar and olive oil. Set aside. Layer tomatoes, mozzarella slices, and basil leaves on a plate or serving tray. Drizzle with vinegar mixture and sprinkle with salt.

Nutritional Information (per serving):
Calories: 289.3
Fat: 24.2 g
Cholesterol: 45.0 mg
Sodium: 440.6 mg
Potassium: 143.5 mg
Carbohydrate: 4.4 g
Protein: 11.8 g

Oven-Roasted Broccoli

Prep Time: 5 minutes
Cook Time: 12 minutes
Yield: 4 servings

Ingredients:
4 c. broccoli florets
2 T. extra virgin olive oil
1 tsp. kosher salt
1/2 tsp. freshly ground black pepper
juice of 1 lemon (optional)

Directions:
Preheat oven to 425°F. Arrange broccoli on a large baking sheet. Drizzle with olive oil and season with salt and pepper. Roast for 10-12 minutes or until the broccoli looks crisp at the edges. Serve with lemon juice. This recipe is equally delicious with 4 c. Brussels sprouts or 4 c. trimmed asparagus spears.

Nutritional Information (per serving):
Calories: 88.3
Fat: 7.3 g
Cholesterol: 0.0 mg
Sodium: 503.9 mg
Potassium: 303.9 mg
Carbohydrate: 5.8 g
Protein: 2.7 g

Grilled Mushroom Skewers

Prep Time: 25 minutes
Cook Time: 15-20 minutes
Yield: 4 servings

Ingredients:
1/4 c. balsamic vinegar
2 T. Worcestershire sauce
2 cloves garlic, minced
2 T. unsalted butter, melted
1/2 tsp. dried thyme
1/2 tsp. dried oregano
1/2 tsp. kosher salt
1/4 tsp. freshly ground black pepper
1 lb. baby bella or button mushrooms
bamboo skewers, soaked

Directions:
In a large bowl, whisk together vinegar, Worcestershire sauce, garlic, and butter. Mix together thyme, oregano, salt, and pepper in a small bowl. Set aside. Add mushrooms and marinate for 20 minutes. While the mushrooms marinate, preheat grill to high heat or oven to 425°F. Slide marinated mushrooms onto skewers and season with thyme mixture. Grill for 8-10 minutes or bake for 15-20 minutes, turning regularly.

Nutritional Information (per serving):
Calories: 94.2
Fat: 5.8 g
Cholesterol: 15.5 mg
Sodium: 387.3 mg
Potassium: 9.5 mg
Carbohydrate: 6.6 g
Protein: 2.7 g

Lemon-Garlic Swiss Chard

Prep Time: 10 minutes
Cook Time: 12 minutes
Yield: 4 servings

Ingredients:
1 T. extra virgin olive oil
1 T. unsalted butter
1 bunch Swiss chard, stems removed and washed
2 cloves garlic, minced
1 c. chicken stock
1/2 tsp. kosher salt
1/4 tsp. freshly ground black pepper
juice of 1 lemon

Directions:
Tear or chop Swiss chard leaves into 2" pieces. Heat oil and butter in a large skillet over medium heat until the butter is melted. Add Swiss chard and cook, stirring as needed, until the Swiss chard is wilted (about 2 minutes). Add the garlic and cook for 2 minutes more. Pour in the chicken stock and cook for 8 minutes. Season with salt, pepper, and lemon juice prior to serving.

Nutritional Information (per serving):
Calories: 89.7
Fat: 6.6 g
Cholesterol: 9.0 mg
Sodium: 715.8 mg
Potassium: 850.4 mg
Carbohydrate: 7.3 mg
Protein: 2.9 g

Bacon-Wrapped Asparagus
Prep Time: 10 minutes
Cook Time: 20 minutes
Yield: 4 servings

Ingredients:
24 asparagus spears, washed and trimmed (about 1 1/2 lb.)
8 slices thick-cut bacon
extra virgin olive oil
kosher salt
freshly ground black pepper

Directions:
Preheat oven to 400°F. Lightly grease a 9x13 casserole pan. Toss asparagus spears in olive oil to coat. Divide asparagus into 8 groups of 3 spears each. Wrap each bundle in 1 slice of bacon. Arrange asparagus bundles in a single layer in the casserole pan and season with salt and pepper. Bake for 15-20 minutes or until the bacon is crispy.

Nutritional Information (per serving):
Calories: 192.4
Fat: 14.7 g
Cholesterol: 25.0 mg
Sodium: 622.0 mg
Potassium: 263.7 mg
Carbohydrate: 4.4 g
Protein: 10.2 g

Creamed Spinach
Prep Time: 10 minutes
Cook Time: 10 minutes
Yield: 8 servings

Ingredients:
4 T. unsalted butter
1 clove garlic, minced
4 c. fresh spinach, washed and chopped
1/2 c. heavy cream
1/4 c. Parmesan cheese
1/2 tsp. kosher salt
1/4 tsp. freshly ground black pepper

Directions:
Melt butter in a large saucepan over medium heat. When the butter is melted, add garlic and spinach. Cook until the spinach has wilted and reduced. Add the cream and cook for 5 minutes. Add the cheese, salt, and pepper. Cook for another 5 minutes or until the creamed spinach has reached the desired consistency.

Nutritional Information (per serving):
Calories: 122.2
Fat: 12.2 g
Cholesterol: 38.4 mg
Sodium: 202.2 mg
Potassium: 18.7 mg
Carbohydrate: 1.5 g
Protein: 2.2 g

Mashed Cauliflower Puree

Prep Time: 5 minutes
Cook Time: 15 minutes
Yield: 6 servings

Ingredients:
1 large head cauliflower, washed and chopped
1/2 c. heavy cream
1/2 c. sour cream
3 T. unsalted butter
1/4 c. sharp cheddar cheese
1/2 tsp. kosher salt
1/4 tsp. freshly ground black pepper

Directions:
Preheat oven to 375°F. Bring a large pot of water to a rolling boil and cook cauliflower for 8 minutes. Strain in a colander and spread the cauliflower out on a large cookie sheet. Bake for 5 minutes. While the cauliflower is baking, bring cream, sour cream, and butter to a simmer. Once the mixture simmers, remove from heat. Combine the cauliflower and cream mixture in a large bowl and puree with an immersion blender. Season with salt and pepper to taste and top with cheese.

Nutritional Information (per serving):
Calories: 213.9
Fat: 18.9 g
Cholesterol: 56.2 mg
Sodium: 250.5 mg
Potassium: 469.6 mg
Carbohydrate: 8.7 g
Protein: 5.0 g

Cobb Salad
Prep Time: 30 minutes
Yield: 6 servings

Ingredients:
1 head romaine lettuce, washed and chopped
1 c. baby spinach, washed
5 hardboiled eggs, peeled and chopped
2 avocados, sliced
8 slices thick-cut bacon
1 c. shredded Colby and Monterey Jack cheese
1 medium tomato, chopped
1 medium cucumber, seeded and chopped

Directions:
Fry bacon in a medium skillet until crisp, reserving grease if desired. Set aside. Fill a large serving bowl with romaine and spinach, tossing to combine. Arrange rows of each topping (eggs, avocado, crumbled bacon, cheese, tomato, and cucumber) to cover the lettuce. Serve immediately. Dress with 1 tablespoon heated bacon grease, equal parts extra virgin olive oil and red wine vinegar, or another low-carbohydrate salad dressing.

Nutritional Information (per serving):
Calories: 317.7
Fat: 24.9 g
Cholesterol: 186.8 mg
Sodium: 417.1 mg
Potassium: 440.9 mg
Carbohydrate: 8.3 g
Protein: 16.0 g

Snacks
Chipotle Cheese Crackers
Prep Time: 30 minutes
Cook Time: 15 minutes
Yield: 25 dozen 1" crackers

Ingredients:
2 1/2 c. almond flour
1/2 tsp. kosher salt
1/2 tsp. baking soda
1/2 tsp. paprika
1/2 tsp. ground chipotle
1 c. shredded cheddar cheese
1/4 c. finely grated Parmesan cheese
3 T. coconut oil
2 eggs, beaten

Directions:
Preheat oven to 350°F. Mix first six ingredients and set aside. In another bowl, beat oil with eggs. Add the egg mixture to the dry ingredients and stir until combined. On a lightly greased surface, roll out the dough to 1/4" thick. Cut into 1" squares using a bench knife, pizza cutter, or greased butter knife and prick each cracker with a fork. Transfer crackers to two parchment-lined baking sheets and sprinkle with Parmesan cheese. Bake for 15 minutes or until the edges of the crackers have browned slightly. Allow the crackers to cool directly on the pan for maximum crispiness.

Nutritional Information (per dozen):
Calories: 102.1
Fat: 9.1 g

Cholesterol: 19.7 mg
Sodium 97.3 mg
Potassium 11.0 mg
Carbohydrate: 2.5 g
Protein: 4.0 g

Kale Chips

Prep Time: 5 minutes
Cook Time: 30 minutes
Yield: 8 servings

Ingredients:
1 head fresh kale
4 T. extra virgin olive oil
1 tsp. kosher salt
fresh cracked pepper, optional

Directions:
Preheat oven to 250°F. Wash kale thoroughly, then chop roughly into pieces the size of a potato chip. Toss kale pieces in olive oil and spread evenly between two half-sheet pans. Sprinkle with salt and pepper (if desired). Bake for 30 minutes, rotating the pans at least once to ensure even cooking.

Nutritional Information (per ½-cup serving):
Calories: 76.5
Fat: 7.3 g
Cholesterol: 0.0 mg
Sodium: 254.4 mg
Potassium: 149.5 mg
Carbohydrate: 3.4 g
Protein: 1.1 g

Deviled Eggs
Prep Time: 10 minutes
Cook Time: 12 minutes
Yield: 8 servings

Ingredients:
12 eggs
1/3 c. mayonnaise
1 tsp. Dijon mustard
2 tsp. pickle juice
1/4 tsp. black pepper
1/4 tsp. smoked paprika

Directions:
Place eggs in a large pot with a lid and cover with cold water. Cook, uncovered, on medium-high heat until boiling. Once the water boils, remove from heat and cover. Let the eggs sit for 12 minutes. Drain immediately and rinse in cold water. Peel the eggs when cool enough to handle.

While the eggs cook, combine mayonnaise, mustard, pickle juice, and spices. Slice eggs in half lengthwise and scoop yolks into a bowl. Set the whites aside. Smash the yolks briefly and then mix with the mayonnaise mixture until fluffy and smooth. If the yolk mixture is too dry, add additional mayonnaise or a splash of plain white vinegar until the desired texture is achieved.

With a spoon or small cookie scoop, fill the hollow of each egg white with a generous scoop of yolk mixture. Serve immediately or cover with plastic wrap and chill until serving.

Nutritional Information (per serving):

Calories: 168.3
Fat: 13.8 g
Cholesterol: 281.5 mg
Sodium: 167.7 mg
Potassium: 106.7 mg
Carbohydrate: 0.7 g
Protein: 9.5 g

Bacon-Wrapped Stuffed Jalapeños

Prep Time: 15 minutes
Cook Time: 25 minutes
Yield: 3 servings

Ingredients:
6 fresh jalapeño peppers
4 oz. cream cheese, softened
1 clove garlic, chopped
1/4 tsp. smoked paprika
1/4 tsp. kosher salt
3 slices thick-cut bacon

Directions:
Preheat oven to 425°F. Combine cream cheese, garlic, paprika, and salt. Set aside. Slice jalapeños lengthwise and remove seeds and membranes. Fill each jalapeño half with cream cheese mixture. Cut each slice of bacon in half and use one half to wrap around each pepper, tucking in the end underneath the jalapeño or securing with toothpicks. Bake for 20-25 minutes or until the bacon is crispy.

Nutritional Information (per serving):
Calories: 189.7
Fat: 17.8 g
Cholesterol: 46.3 mg
Sodium: 422.4 mg
Potassium: 120.3 mg
Carbohydrate: 3.6 g
Protein: 5.3 g

Ham and Cheese Pickle Pinwheel Roll Ups

Prep Time: 15 minutes
Yield: 20 servings

Ingredients:
20 slices smoked deli ham
8 oz. cream cheese, softened
20 slices Swiss cheese
20 small sweet pickles

Directions:
Spread a thin layer of cream cheese on each slice of ham. Center a slice of swiss cheese on each slice of ham. Place a sweet pickle at the end of each ham and cheese stack. Roll tightly. Slice each roll into 3 even slices. Serve chilled.

Nutritional Information (per each 3 pinwheels):
Calories: 141.4
Fat: 9.3 g
Cholesterol: 39.9 mg
Sodium: 344.4 mg
Potassium: 20.4 mg
Carbohydrate: 5.5 g
Protein: 8.4 g

Chocolate Chip Protein Bites

Prep Time: 30 minutes
Chill Time: 1 hour
Yield: 40 bites

Ingredients:
1 c. raw almonds
1 c. raw cashews
4 c. shredded coconut, unsweetened
1/2 c. coconut oil
1 2/3 c. natural peanut butter
1/2 c. chia seeds
1/2 c. flax seeds
1/2 c. dark chocolate chips, chopped

Directions:
Toast nuts, seeds, and coconut on a parchment-lined baking sheet for 10-12 minutes in a 300°F oven. Once the nut-and-seed mixture has cooled slightly, pulse the mixture in a food processor 4-5 times. In a large bowl, combine coconut oil and peanut butter. Stir in the nut-and-seed mixture until combined. Stir in the chocolate chips.

Scoop the mixture 1 tablespoon at a time and roll into packed balls. It will be easier to roll the balls if your hands are wet and the mixture is slightly chilled. Place the protein bites on a parchment-lined baking sheet and chill thoroughly.

Nutritional Information (per bite):
Calories: 211.4
Fat: 19.0 g
Cholesterol: 0.0 mg

Sodium: 52.0 mg
Potassium: 62.3 mg
Carbohydrate: 9.5 g
Protein: 5.0 g

Pantry Staples
Homemade Mayonnaise
Prep Time: 10 minutes
Yield: 1 1/4 cup

Ingredients:
1 egg yolk
1 tsp. yellow mustard
1/2 tsp. kosher salt
2 tsp. apple cider vinegar
1 T. lemon juice
1 c. avocado oil

Directions:
In a small bowl, combine vinegar and lemon juice and set aside. Put egg yolk, mustard, and salt in a blender or food processor and pulse until combined. Add half of the vinegar/lemon juice mixture to the blender. With the blender on low, slowly pour 1/2 cup oil in through the lid. It is very important to pour the oil in slowly so that the mayonnaise can emulsify properly. Once half the oil is incorporated, drizzle in the remaining vinegar and lemon juice. Add the remaining 1/2 cup oil by slowly pouring it into the mixture while the blender or food processor continues to whip the mayonnaise. Continue blending until the mixture is thick. Any light-tasting oil can be used in this recipe.

Nutritional Information (per tablespoon):
Calories: 106.9
Fat: 11.4 g
Cholesterol: 9.2 mg
Sodium: 51.2 mg
Potassium: 1.6 mg

Carbohydrate: 0.0 g
Protein: 0.1 g

Bone Broth
Prep Time: 5 minutes
Cook Time: 24+ hours
Yield: varies

Ingredients:
3-4 pounds soup bones or bone-in scraps
6 ribs celery, chopped
4 carrots, chopped
2 onions, quartered
6 cloves of garlic, peeled
3 bay leaves
1 bunch herb stems (thyme, parsley, rosemary, etc.)
2 T. apple cider vinegar
1-2 gallons water

Directions:
If the bones are not from a previous meal, roast the bones or scraps at 400°F for 45 minutes or until fragrant. If the bones and scraps are left from a previously cooked dish, skip this step. Put soup bones or scraps in a large stock pot and cover with water and vinegar. Bring the water to a boil, then reduce the heat until just high enough to maintain a low simmer. Periodically skim foam and impurities from the top of the pot for the first hour. Simmer for 12-48 hours. The longer it simmers, the more developed the flavors will be in the final broth. Add more water if needed to keep the bones completely covered.

After at least 12 hours, add the vegetables and herbs. Simmer for an additional 8-12 hours. Use a fine-meshed sieve to strain the broth into a large bowl that has been placed on ice. Discard the solids. For a clearer broth, strain a second time through cheesecloth to remove any impurities. Serve immediately or ladle broth into jars for storing in the refrigerator, freezing, or canning.

Nutritional Information (per 8 oz. serving):

Specifics will vary, depending on the bones and aromatics used in making each batch of bone broth. The following is for beef bone broth made with grass-fed beef soup bones and garlic.

Calories: 69.2
Fat: 4.0 g
Cholesterol: 18.1 mg
Sodium: 232.8 mg
Potassium: 10.4 mg
Carbohydrate: 0.8 g
Protein: 6.4 g

Nut and Seed Cereal Mix
Prep Time: 5 minutes
Yield: 4 cups mix

Ingredients:
1 c. flax seed meal
1/2 c. oat bran
1/2 c. almonds, ground
1/2 c. pecans, ground
1/2 c. sunflower seeds, ground
1 c. vanilla protein powder

Directions:
Mix all ingredients. Store in a large container with a lid in a cool, dry place. To make the cereal, combine 1/4 cup mix with 1/2 cup boiling water. Let sit covered for 5 minutes and serve with a splash of heavy cream.

Nutritional Information (per serving):
Calories: 153.8
Fat: 8.4 g
Cholesterol: 7.5 mg
Sodium: 75.2 mg
Potassium: 145.0 mg
Carbohydrate: 6.4 g
Protein: 14.5 g

Cilantro-Lime Compound Butter
Prep Time: 5 minutes
Chill Time: 4 hours
Yield: 1/2 cup

Ingredients:
1/2 c. unsalted butter, softened
2 T. lime juice
1 clove garlic, minced
2 T. cilantro leaves, minced

Directions:
Combine all ingredients in a small bowl or food processor. Spoon mixture onto a long piece of plastic wrap or parchment paper. Roll tightly and chill 3-4 hours. To use, top grilled chicken, fish, or vegetables with a thick slice. The cilantro and lime juice can be substituted for lemon juice or vinegar and any herb to suit the meal or preference of the guests. Substituting half the butter for smashed avocado is another easy keto-friendly variation.

Nutritional Information (per tablespoon):
Calories: 103.7
Fat: 11.5 g
Cholesterol: 31.1 mg
Sodium: 1.8 mg
Potassium: 16.4 mg
Carbohydrate: 0.1 g
Protein: 0.1 g

Chapter 8 Takeaways

1. Ketogenic recipes can be delicious and varied.

2. You can still eat well-rounded and tasty meals on a ketogenic diet.

3. Many other recipes can be adapted to a ketogenic diet using the same principles outlined in these recipes.

4. Any of the recipes that call for sugar-free flavoring syrup or protein powder can be easily changed from vanilla to chocolate or any other flavor. Simply replace the vanilla protein powder or vanilla flavoring with the flavor of your choice.

One Last Thought

Whether you are looking to lose weight, improve your mental clarity, or lower your blood sugar, a ketogenic diet has something to offer everyone willing to put in the work. Specifics vary from person to person, but a ketogenic diet is a great way to get consistent, long-term results. By forcing your body to derive energy from fat, you will break your reliance on carbohydrates and sugars and take advantage of the natural metabolic process known as ketosis.

You CAN find more energy and confidence now.

With the help of the chapters in this book, you can transition to a ketogenic diet without spending a fortune. The information provided will help you be confident in the process and aware of any risk factors. A ketogenic diet is not a fad diet. It does not lend itself to half-hearted commitment, but if you are willing to go against the grain and remove carbohydrates from your diet, you will see results. Using the resources, recipes, and 8-week meal plan, you are now ready to take the first step toward a thinner, healthier you.

Can You Help?

I'd love to hear your opinion about my book. In the world of book publishing, there are few things more valuable than honest reviews from a wide variety of readers.

Your review will help other readers find out if my book is for them. It will also help me reach more readers by increasing the visibility of my book.

You can leave your reviews here.

Resources Cited

Made in the USA
Middletown, DE
13 December 2016